The
Moon
Is
Broken

OTHER BOOKS BY ELEANOR CRAIG

P.S. Your Not Listening (1971)

1-2-3: The Story of Matt, a Feral Child (1978)

If We Could Hear the Grass Grow (1983)

The Moon Is Broken

A Mother's True Story

Eleanor Craig

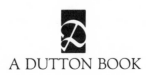

A DUTTON BOOK

DUTTON
Published by the Penguin Group
Penguin Books USA Inc., 375 Hudson Street,
New York, New York 10014, U.S.A.
Penguin Books Ltd, 27 Wrights Lane, London W8 5TZ, England
Penguin Books Australia Ltd, Ringwood, Victoria, Australia
Penguin Books Canada Ltd, 10 Alcorn Avenue,
Toronto, Ontario, Canada M4V 3B2
Penguin Books (N.Z.) Ltd, 182-190 Wairau Road, Auckland 10, New Zealand

Penguin Books Ltd, Registered Offices:
Harmondsworth, Middlesex, England

First published by Dutton, an imprint of New American Library,
a division of Penguin Books USA Inc.
Distributed in Canada by McClelland & Stewart Inc.

First Printing, February, 1992
10 9 8 7 6 5 4 3 2 1

 REGISTERED TRADEMARK—MARCA REGISTRADA

Library of Congress Cataloging-in-Publication Data
Craig, Eleanor.
   The moon is broken : a mother's story / Eleanor Craig.
      p. cm.
ISBN 0-525-93401-4
1. Craig, Ann—Mental health. 2. Mentally ill—United States—Biography. 3. Craig, Ann—
Health. 4. AIDS (Disease)—Patients—United States—Biography. 5. Craig, Eleanor—
Family. 6. Mothers and daughters—United States—Case studies. 7. Psychotherapists—
United States—Biography. I. Title.
RC464.C69C73 1992
616.89'0092—dc20
[B]   91-20292
                                                                                      CIP

Printed in the United States of America
Set in Goudy Old Style
Designed by Eve L. Kirch

This book is dedicated to all who seek the serenity to
accept the things they cannot change,
the courage to change the things they can,
and the wisdom to know the difference.

Acknowledgments

With deepest appreciation to my husband Paul, to my family, and to friends—both mine and Ann's—for accepting my need to write this book, and for their understanding when the writing usurped time I would have liked to spend with them.

Thanks to Alexia Dorszynski, Senior Editor at Dutton, for her insight, talent, and ever-available encouragement.

Years of thanks to my agent, Don Congdon, for generous input, readings and re-readings, and for having faith in me even when my own faith wavered.

*The
Moon
Is
Broken*

Prologue

It is hard to let go of hopes for a child. What had happened to Annie, I asked myself time and again. Was it her involvement in the drug culture of the sixties that left my daughter teetering at the brink of what she called "a terrible black abyss," unable to pursue becoming the anthropologist she dreamed of being, unable even to finish her final thesis at Brown University? I only knew that I, a family therapist with many years of clinical experience, could not draw on any professional objectivity that enabled me to help her.

The Moon Is Broken is the story of our mother-daughter struggle. I began the writing for myself, hoping that contact with her friends in New York would enable me to fit together the pieces I had yet to understand.

"I thought perhaps I would not hear from you again," her friend Randy told me. "I cringe remembering the incessantly ringing telephone we both left unanswered for fear it was someone in the family who might remind us of who we really were."

The motivation to expand my notes into a book came from finding in Ann's own writings that her perspective differed greatly from mine. From that discovery on, I felt we were co-authors and proceeded with the hope that our experience—hers, mine, and our family's—might be of value to others.

Snapshots

Even as a little child, Annie was both dramatic and caring. The youngest and the smallest in her kindergarten Christmas pageant, it was she who sang the loudest and then nudged all the bigger children, reminding them to bow.

Annie was eleven the time she took five-year-old Billy skating on shallow Mill Pond and he fell through the ice. I was standing at the kitchen window when I saw them coming home—Annie carrying her shivering little brother on her back, her mittens on his feet.

Throughout her school years she produced and acted in the plays she wrote. Her theme was resolution to injustice, from converting the playground bully to a good kid to negotiating peace in Northern Ireland. In eighth grade Ann auditioned for a community theater production. It was a part she wanted more than any other.

February 1, 1966

Dear Diary,

Today was try-outs for the play. All day long I felt so nervous that I couldn't eat. But guess what! Mr. Gallagher chose me. Je m'appelle Ann Frank!

Tonight I am reading her diary. She was exactly my age when she wrote it. How could Ann Frank live in such frightening circumstances and still hold on to such high ideals?

March 17, 1966

Happy Saint Patrick's Day. Everything I wore today was green. Mr. Gallagher teased me at rehearsal. He said, "I didn't know you were Italian."

And I sure got teased by the cast about the scene where I get kissed by Peter, even though we just pretended. I used to think that teasing was a way of being friendly. Now I think that people ought to look for kinder ways.

April 25, 1966

Oh, but I am sooo happy. I hate to sound like a braggart but everyone said we were great. I hope that every person in the theater left caring about who Ann Frank was. Someday I'd like to be a writer. Even though she died, Ann Frank's words will always survive.

Well, au revoir, dear Diary

P.S. I didn't mind kissing Peter.

I gave Ann the picture poster of my mother, who died before her grandchildren were born. MARIE LOUISE O'BRIEN, it read, STARRING IN *Peg O' My Heart*. I had seen the resemblance so clearly as I watched my child onstage. The same quick, deliberate gestures, the same dark wavy hair with auburn highlights, the same high cheekbones and deepset eyes.

Ann taped the poster to her bedroom mirror. "After I finish working as an anthropologist in Africa," she said, "I'll be an actress, like my grandma. And then a writer." She smiled at me. "I don't want to be afraid to try a lot of different life-styles. If Anne Frank could believe in people, it should be easy for me. Remember how she said 'In spite of everything, I still believe that people are really good at heart'?"

As Ann repeated the words, I was swept with a current of tenderness and love for my firstborn.

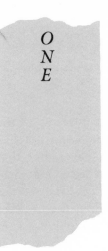

On a High with Annie

"When are you coming home?" I asked.

"Soon," she said, but I could hear the uncertainty in my daughter's voice. "As—uh—as soon as I finish my senior thesis. I—uh—I have to get it in, Ma. I just can't come home until I finish."

I hadn't looked at the 1975 college calendar to determine a specific date, but I had assumed that Ann would return from college as soon as spring term ended. Then, on my way home from work at the Child Guidance Clinic, I stopped to pick up vegetables at Grand Union, and there was Annie's classmate, Steven Brophy. He raised his eyebrows when I asked what he was doing buying apples in Connecticut. "Ann isn't home yet? Our anthropology exams ended over a week ago."

I got the vegetable casserole in the oven before I called her, expecting to hear that all was well and she had chosen to stay for the fun of having postsemester freedom with friends, or perhaps to paint her small off-campus apartment.

It worried me, the flat halting delivery of words from a daughter whose voice was usually so enthusiastic.

"Annie, you sound like something's wrong. Anything I could do to help?"

"Oh, Ma, I—uh—I just cannot get away, but if you would come to Providence—I-I sure could use a Mamma visit."

I made the calls necessary to cancel my appointments at the clinic for that next day, the tenth day of June. I did not like having to postpone a therapy session for any client, but that night I felt most concerned about not seeing Eileen Driscoll, a sixteen-year-old victim of her father's alcoholic rages. Her mother enabled his behavior by pleading with the children not to make him angry. Eileen, the oldest, had turned her anger inward, finally overdosing on aspirin. She became my patient upon her release from the hospital. The pretty girl sat silent and withdrawn the first two times we met; it was only the previous week that she had finally begun to open up about her overwhelming sense of helplessness and despair.

When I said I had to postpone our appointment, Eileen said it was okay. But her voice was flat. Flat, the way my own daughter's had sounded.

I left Tuesday morning without waking my husband. Bill had been up most of the night, struggling with an overdue manuscript. He got to bed as my alarm clock sounded 6:00 A.M.

Our fifteen-year-old son Billy had an early-morning orchestra rehearsal. I dropped him and his big string bass at Staples High School, then took the youngest of my four, thirteen-year-old Ellen, to the junior high.

Heading north on Interstate 95, I felt a mounting anxiety about what might be so upsetting to Ann. I remembered the relief, four years before, when we first drove her to Brown, putting distance between her and the friends she had made her senior year in high school—a group of artists and musicians in their early twenties who lived communally, performing concerts and tie-dying T-shirts for income.

Bill and I had never been concerned before about our eldest child's friends. At the start of her junior year in high school, our family had moved to Germany for a year, where Bill was to research a book on the battle of Stalingrad. All four children attended the International School at Oberursal. There Ann's social life had centered on a single relationship, a tender first romance. But Eric and his family returned to their home in Canada, we moved back to Connecticut, and gradually, as their correspondence tapered off, she began to spend free time with the tie-dyers. Like them, she took a leadership role in silent vigils and ardent marches protesting U.S. involvement in Vietnam.

She was still a splendid student, and still the supportive daughter, always ready with excellent editorial suggestions when she read my manuscripts. But she avoided family outings, and our mother-daughter shopping trips, which once had been such special fun, fell by the wayside. She and her father argued about her choice of bed jackets for blouses, "indecent" jeans, and the time she spent with "hippies." Bill and I, realizing how much Ann had changed, warned her against drug use, though we had no evidence to support our fears.

On my way to work one October morning, I was frustrated to find myself caught in much heavier than normal traffic. A group of demonstrators, holding placards, were blocking off the downtown bridge. Others fanned out through the lines of honking cars to distribute leaflets. The driver in the car ahead yelled, "Get the hell away from me, you little commie bastard."

The demonstrator came toward my car. I did not look up until she said, "Hello, Ma."

"Annie! I thought you went to school."

"This is more important. See you later, Ma," she said, thrusting a piece of paper through my window and heading for another car. It read:

AFTER NINE YEARS OF WAR IN VIETNAM
37,000 AMERICANS
AND HUNDREDS OF THOUSANDS OF VIETNAMESE ARE DEAD
THE VICTIMS OF U.S. IMPERIALISM
LEAVE THE CARES OF THE CITY BEHIND
GET AWAY FROM IT ALL

COME TO FABULOUS FORT DIX
SUNDAY OCTOBER 12th

In springtime, just before her high school graduation, Ann went for a swim at a nearby pond. Two hours later I turned off the vacuum cleaner to take a phone call. "Mrs. Craig? Officer Sullivan here. You have a daughter Ann Marie Craig? We've got her at the station. Possession of marijuana. You folks can bail her out if you want."

Before her trial date, Ann explained to the lawyer that an off-duty policeman had spotted her and five tie-dyer friends passing a "suspicious-looking pipe" as they picnicked by the pond. "I wasn't 'in possession.' The one who brought it simply offered it around. But they sent six police cars to pick up six terrified pacifists, handcuffed each of us, and took us off in our bathing suits, saying our towels and robes had to be held for 'evidence.' "

At her trial, Bill and I heard the judge's sentence—one year on probation—as reinforcement to our warnings. We hoped that she did also.

Once we helped her move into her dormitory at Brown I felt much more comfortable, knowing she was distanced from the tie-dyer friends—until the night the eleven o'clock news ran a special feature on campus demonstrations. Suddenly Bill and I spotted our daughter in the front of the crowd that had gathered on the steps of the administration building, protecting minority students who had taken over inside.

It was midnight when I finally reached her by phone. She had just returned to her room to get a coat. I said, "Listen to me, Ann. Please do not go back there if you think there will be trouble."

"But, Mother, that's just when we have to be there—if there's trouble."

The last time I had driven to Brown, also in response to her asking for a "Mamma visit," Ann told me she would not be able to graduate and would have to return in September. I remembered her elaborate explanation about the points for advanced placement courses she had taken in high school not being counted. It was not like Ann to be uncertain about credits.

Her father and I were anxious that she finish. Our writing incomes were sporadic; my salary at the clinic covered only basics. Richard, our second oldest, had two years left at Southern Connecticut, and then there would be college fees for Billy and for Ellen two years later.

Ann had already taken extra time getting through. She and her classmate Tim had been in Africa from June of 1974 through January of 1975, each researching material for the senior thesis. Together they traveled by foot, bus, and train, moving from Egypt down the African east coast. For Tim, the journey centered on the history of the slave trade; Ann's topic was "The Evolving Roles of Witchcraft and Religion in Contemporary African Culture."

Ann arrived at home wearing a blue batik gown, her head wrapped in a conical turban of the same bright cloth. Her sunburned nose was flecked with freckles, her cheeks rounder than when she left—more like a little girl's than a college senior's.

Her green canvas backpack bulged with ancient-looking jewelry from Egypt, black clay religious figures sculpted by Ethiopian Jews, and beautiful hardwood carvings from Nairobi. But more precious than any piece of artwork were the three worn leather diaries in which she had recorded the details of the days she spent with witch doctors in sophisticated cities and primitive villages.

On a dark night, under a crescent moon, my mentor, the village witch doctor, offered to initiate me into the first stage of witchcraft. Pointing, he offered the space between my teeth as evidence of my ability to extend good fortune to others. What the orthodontist failed to correct had suddenly become my greatest asset! As thirty villagers sat around the embers of a brush fire, he took a knife and cut a small X on the palm of my hand. Before I could prevent it he took a burning ember and placed it on the wound. It was terribly sore, but the pain entitled me to a black leather witch doctor's bag, containing horns, gourds, and leather sacks with herbs and powders, each for a specific purpose.

(DIARY ENTRY)

I had made no secret of my uneasiness about her interest in witchcraft. I remembered how Ann laughed at my concern. "What you call my 'risk taking,' Ma, is really my curiosity," she said. The two-hour drive had provided me the thinking time to reflect that I would be relieved to have her finish the thesis and leave the subject of witchcraft behind.

I drove up the familiar hill to Thayer Street, past the campus dormitories where Ann had stayed so briefly. Early into her freshman year Ann had waged a strident campaign to move off-campus to her own "space"—two rooms in a rambling wooden house on Charles Field Road.

I knocked on her door several times; then, getting no response, I began to head for the end of the hallway, to check the single bathroom that served the three apartments. I jumped as Ann's door suddenly creaked open and Ann, in an old silk paisley robe, murmured, "Sorry, Ma. I only got to sleep a little while ago."

She leaned into my shoulder. I wrapped my arms around her, but her own arms remained at her sides. "How come, dear?" I tried to run my hand through her long thick hair but found my fingers caught in the kind of early-morning tangles she woke up with as a little girl.

"Just go on in, Ma, I'll be more awake in a minute," she said. Then, toothbrush and towel in hand, Ann went off to the bathroom.

I sat on the paisley shawl she liked to drape on her bed, and looked around the room. Even with the curtains partially drawn, I could see that something was very wrong. There had to be at least a hundred books—each loaded with cards and papers—stacked on the table, chairs, and up against the wall. Last time I had visited there had been no mention, nor any sign in the room, of what now seemed so apparent—she was having a very difficult time getting organized.

Returning from the bathroom, she leaned into the little mirror above the kitchen sink to brush thick black mascara on her lashes.

"Your room looks like Dad's office," I said watching her. "Only he is writing a four-hundred-page book. Annie, how can you possibly integrate all this, with all the notes in your diaries, into a single report? You must feel absolutely swamped. Couldn't you narrow your focus?"

She wheeled and glared, her look clearly intended to silence me. "Ma, I do not want suggestions. I know what I have to do." She turned back to the mirror and used her middle finger to smooth a shiny balm onto her generous lips.

Then she sat down on the bed beside me, her arm around my shoulder. "Remember my friend Greg, Ma? The fellow finishing his masters in English lit? Well, he's the one in trouble. He knows that you're a therapist and he was so relieved when I told him you might see him. Could we take him out to breakfast—just for an hour or so?"

Although I knew she wanted to shift my attention away from herself, I agreed to see Greg. After I took them to breakfast, I reasoned, she might be ready to talk.

While we waited for her friend, Ann took me on our ritual visit to her elderly neighbors. Gracious, dotty Mr. Carbone greeted Ann by pinching her cheeks. "Annie, Annie," he said, clasping her hand in both of his and smiling adoringly. Mrs. Carbone peered over her husband's shoulder.

"I brought my mamma to say hello. She wants to know how Tweetie is doing, don't you, Ma?"

"Tweetie don't sing for no strangers," Mrs. Carbone snapped, yanking Mr. Carbone by the collar.

"Come back soon, Ann," he called through the door.

"Glory be to God, Ann, it's your mither!" Miss Cahill had a single room across the hall. "And you two looking so much alike. Well, come right in now, won't ya, and have a touch of sherry."

"Another time," Ann smiled. "Mom and I are going out to breakfast."

"Well, may the Blessed Virgin Mary bless you both now." Miss Cahill shut the door.

Greg finally arrived, in a T-shirt with a sunburst of sequins and jeans with more holes than Ann's. Breakfast turned into lunch, as Greg described his parents' impending divorce, and how the trauma had rendered him unable either to take his final exams or to hold on to his girlfriend.

"Sandy turned to a more supportive relationship with a woman," he said. After wolfing down a second nutburger, Greg shook my hand, promising to accept my suggestion to seek on-going counseling.

"That was great, Ma." My daughter hugged me as we left the restaurant. "He's been so despairing. I was really worried. Gosh," she paused to look at the cloudless sky, "it's such a glorious day. Could we drive over to the Plymouth Airport? I'll show you the gliders I've been flying. I'd love to introduce you to Ron, my instructor."

Again I found myself believing that time together on her terms would make it easier to talk about her paper later. Driving through the flowering countryside, I felt I had made the right decision. Like her old enthusiasic self, Ann began reciting funny stories.

"My first lesson with Ron started off so gently, Mom. 'Okay now, honey, it's time to put the flaps down. I said *now!* Listen you stupid kid, put down the fucking flaps.' "

"Annie," I laughed, "Ron's vocabulary is a little stronger, but he still sounds like Grandpa teaching me to drive."

Ron, a stocky fellow in a leather jacket, came out of the small terminal to greet her with a bear hug. "Annie, baby! Just in time! Got me a package to deliver over to the Vineyard. How'd you like to copilot my Cessna?"

I, who deliberately avoided travel in small planes, watched in nervous excitement from the seat behind as Ron and Ann went down the preflight checklist.

The plane was climbing when Ron called, "Okay, your turn to fly her, girl!" And Ann took the controls.

Remembering a favorite poem, I surrendered to the beauty of the sky and sparkling ocean.

Oh, I have slipped the surly bonds of earth
And danced the sky on laughter-silvered wings . . .

The sun was setting as we climbed out of the cockpit back at Plymouth Airport. "If I were younger I'd marry this girl," Ron said as he hugged her.

Ann and I ran across the field giggling like school kids, our arms around each other.

"Wasn't that great, Ma?"

"Oh, it was wonderful, Annie!"

On the ride back to Rhode Island I asked her what she thought the problem was with her writing. Ann looked straight ahead for a moment. I wasn't sure she would answer. Then she said, "You're right, Ma, I've got to narrow the focus. Maybe someday I'll be able to use the rest of the material in a book. I don't want you to worry. I'll be finished in a week or so. Then I'll come home and get a summer job."

We kissed good-bye in front of her apartment.

By 8:00 P.M. I was back on the thruway hemmed in by tractor-trailers but relieved by her promise and exhilarated by our flight. I told myself I had been foolish to worry. Ann had always been too hard on herself about schoolwork, but she had always gotten it done.

Bill got up from his desk when I drove in at eleven. "How did it go?"

I told him about the flight and then how she had buried herself in research.

"I know how that feels," he said.

We split a tuna sandwich. On the way upstairs to our room I said, "It's odd how anxious I felt about her when I left this morning. Now I end the day feeling as if I've been on some kind of high with Annie."

At last you switch into panic gear—precipitated by lack of confidence in your own ability to handle the work, thus fearful of the work itself. You lose perspective, begin to be unable to perceive reasonable limitations to that which is required of you. Sense of desperate drive to goals of superlativeness that would render you utterly beyond reproach. Therefore SAFE.

How can you be vulnerable—if you've done everything? Yet the expectation that perfection is in any way achievable is in itself a danger.

Conclusion: No way to avoid the peril.

(DIARY ENTRY, JUNE 10, 1975)

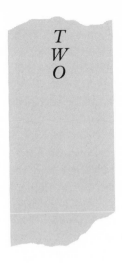

Finding Out

June was a busy month at the clinic—time to reassess the children who had been in special education classes and to help the schools plan placements for the fall. There were so many more options now for nonretarded kids with special needs than had existed in 1960, when I had taught the first class for "socially and emotionally maladjusted children." Back then, neither the testing materials nor the vocabulary to identify attention deficit disorder and dyslexia existed.

Learning-disabled students were inappropriately grouped with the most emotionally troubled, "acting-out," and severely withdrawn children. The first parents' organization to advocate in behalf of those who would later be described as dyslexic called itself the Association for Brain-Injured Children, only later switching to the less pejorative title of the Association for Children with Learning Disabilities.

Workdays were long. At home every evening, keeping myself alert with cup after cup of coffee, I tried to push ahead with the writing of my second book, the case study of a boy with whom I worked whose behavior was so bizarre that the psychiatrist at our clinic labeled him "a feral child"—as wild as if raised by animals. My first book, *P.S. Your Not Listening*, had received wonderful reviews, and it was frightening to attempt to match its success. But I had to try.

For me, writing was like solving a complex yet compelling puzzle—the task of mentally sorting through hundreds of work hours to pinpoint moments best able to describe the behaviors of a single troubled child. And only writing, the physical putting down on paper of those experiences, afforded me the clearing and renewal to continue work I both loved and so often found depleting. Ideally, describing the plight of abused and neglected children would enable those whose work was unrelated to understand the need for special educational and therapeutic programs.

But the price was high. Finding time to write forced me to be less available to my family, who understood, and to friends, many of whom did not. Someday, I told myself, I would do nothing but write. Over the years as both teacher and therapist I had collected cartons of notes, a store large enough for a lifetime. But I could not take the risk of such uncertain income. Writing had to be an evening and weekend pursuit.

One Friday night, while I spread pages on the kitchen table and Richard, Billy, and Ellen were loading up the dishwasher, Billy commented that he had been surprised when I had told him Ann was having trouble with her thesis. Ellen agreed. She thought of schoolwork as coming easily to her sister.

The phone rang.

"I'm sorry I've been out of touch, Ma," Ann sounded shaky. "I guess I've had it. Both mentally and physically I'm exhausted. But the mental part is the worst."

I felt my heart race. "Let me bring you home," I said, fearing she would protest. But she did not resist. "Just rest as much as you can tonight. I'll be there in the morning."

Richard offered to drive. When we got to her apartment, we found the door ajar. Ann was sitting in her bathrobe staring at a jumbled splay of papers. She said she had been up all night. She rested her head on the table while we packed up her books, filled boxes with her notes, unloaded her jammed-up closet, and carried carton after carton down the stairs. Rich and I returned scores of borrowed books to the campus library. Ann gazed blankly from the window of the car. She slept all the way home, curled up like a baby.

Over the next few days, Annie's spirits lifted. I shared her excitement when she got a job as stage manager at the Old Mill Summer Theatre. Most weekends, she took the train to Springfield, Massachusetts, to be with her friend Tim. One Saturday he came to our house instead. That night their angry voices carried from the front hallway to my upstairs bedroom.

"I can't tolerate it," Tim said. "It feels like emotional blackmail to know and not be able to help you."

"I support you unconditionally," Ann said. "I have a right to expect you to do the same for me."

"But Ann, the situations are not comparable."

Someone slammed the door. Tim's footsteps faded down the road.

I would not pretend I hadn't heard them. I knocked at her bedroom door. "Are you okay, Ann?"

She peeked out and I saw that she'd been crying. "Don't worry, Ma. I made the mistake of telling Tim something he couldn't handle. The director at the theater has been asking me out."

She began to close the door.

"Whoa, Annie, it sounded more serious than that—"

"You don't think that's serious to Tim, Ma? What did you think it was about?" she demanded. "Did you think poor Ann must be pregnant? Well, I'm not." She closed the door.

> *Foolish pride*
> *Lovers tangled in combat*
> *No one speaks*
> *We fear love more than war*
> *Only sound is my heart*
> *Slowly breaking*
> *Leave me now as I've left you before*
>
> (DIARY ENTRY, AUGUST 1975)

Tim's visits became shorter and less frequent. In mid-August their intense three-year relationship, highlighted by their African trek, had cooled. Ann started dating the director. But as September approached she began expressing great anxiety about her unfinished paper and having to return to school. I talked to her about getting some help, perhaps from a family therapist. That was my orientation, and I felt it made sense for Ann's difficulty to be seen in that context.

She did not resist the idea of therapy, but she insisted on going alone. "I'm twenty-two years old," she said. "My problems concern my future. That's mine to face alone. I will not go with the family."

Understandably enough, she did not want to work with anyone who knew me. My friend Shirley Sarkin, chief social worker for the schools, made several recommendations. Ann spoke by phone to three of the people Shirley suggested and made an appointment with a Dr. Gerald Robbins.

Ann liked the psychiatrist and began to see him weekly. She did not talk about their meetings.

The last Sunday in August, Ann spent the day in her room. Late that afternoon I thought I heard a muffled cry.

"Are you all right?" I stood at her door. Silence. Frightening silence. I turned the knob and entered.

"I don't want anyone in here, and that includes you," she said.

I could hardly believe it. Ann's voice was coming from the closet. She was hiding like a child.

"Annie," I said, "I'm here to help you."

"Then get out of my room."

"Not until I see you." Suddenly I had horrifying images of her holding a rope or a knife.

"If I come out," she said, "you must promise to leave."

Her body was shaking. She took tiny steps across the room and let me ease her into bed.

It was a sweltering night, but Ann was wearing a long-sleeved sweater. I tried to remove it, but she pushed my hands away and wrapped herself in her quilt.

I sat by her bed. "What is it, Annie? What in God's name is it? Are you ill?"

"I don't know, Ma. I've been having violent nightmares. They leave me feeling hopeless and empty, as though I'm standing at the brink of a deep black pit that could suck me in."

I felt frightened, yet wanted to reassure her. "I'm here, dear. And Dr. Robbins will help you too. Nothing matters but your health now."

Ann was almost asleep when she reached out for my hand. "Please don't worry, Mamma."

After her next appointment, Dr. Robbins called to ask that Bill and I come in with Ann. We set the meeting for the day after Bill was due home from what he hoped would be his final research trip for the Stalingrad book. But he returned from Russia unhappy that an interview he had not been able to schedule would further delay the delivery of his manuscript. I found it hard to add to his worries by telling him Ann seemed more troubled.

The next day's meeting with Dr. Robbins began with the psychiatrist turning to Ann. "I'd like you to tell your parents just how badly you have felt," he said.

She turned away. "They do not need to know."

"I cannot agree with that," he persisted. "I told you this is something your parents have a right to know."

Ann bit her lip. He waited.

"Very well then, I will help you."

I held my breath, afraid to listen.

"Ann is very hard on herself," the psychiatrist began. "She sees her inability to finish her paper as a weakness. In a very complex kind of self-punishment, Ann cut herself on her arms several times during spring semester. She did this again at home in her closet just last Sunday night."

Sunday night. In her closet. When I was filled with fear that she might be capable of hurting herself. So that was why she wore the long-sleeved sweater. I had the nauseous feeling of falling from a railless balcony and tumbling slowly through space.

Ann rose from her chair and began to pace. She argued with the doctor, insisting that her cuts were foolish, superficial attempts to release unbearable tension. "I told you it was my *solution*," she said, wringing her hands. "Why do you call it a problem?"

"I have spoken to Ann about hospitalization," the doctor said.

"No!" Ann fled from the office. Bill and I leaped from the couch to stop her. I was terrified. I thought I had seen a razor blade in her hand.

"Wait," Dr. Robbins said to me. "Let her father go. I need to sign an admission order. Take her to the emergency room." He signed a form and handed it to me.

Bill found Ann crouched behind a snow fence. He put her between us in the car. I drove to the hospital.

The turbaned, bearded psychiatric resident who examined Ann found Bill and me in the waiting room. "In spite of your fears, your daughter is carrying no dangerous object. She is three points oriented; she is well aware of her name, the date, and where she is at the moment. I therefore see no cause for involuntary hospitalization. Of course, I see that she has scars on her arm, but these must be looked upon as gestures. Unless your daughter signs a voluntary commitment paper, which she is unwilling to do, I cannot commit her. I'm sorry."

"But her own psychiatrist signed her in," Bill said, holding out Dr. Robbins's paper, "for her own protection."

"I cannot commit her," the resident repeated and turned away.

Refusing to accept his verdict, Bill headed for the pay phone to enlist more help from Dr. Robbins. But he could only suggest that we drive to another hospital and try to get her admitted.

"Could I make a bargain with you, Dad and Mom?" Ann spoke calmly as we started. "I will not commit myself—not tonight. But if you two will just give me time to talk to Dr. Robbins about some places he suggested, I promise to go to whatever hospital seems the best the day after my birthday." Her proposal meant a wait of almost two months.

Bill and I conferred in her presence. We did not want to drive from one hospital to another, nor did she any longer look like a candidate for involuntary admission. We really had no choice but to trust her. We took her home on her promise not to hurt herself again.

At times the wait was terrifying for me. Sometimes when Ann was in her room or in the bathroom I would listen at the door, haunted by dark images of her harming herself. There were nights when she wanted to talk for hours, expressing fears of becoming lost in a black abyss. The painful talks were often followed by periods of aloofness.

Dr. Robbins agreed with Ann's choice of place for treatment: Austen Riggs Center in Stockbridge, Massachusetts, one of the few psychoanalytic residential facilities in the country. He felt that Ann's own insight and capacity for understanding made the psychoanalytic approach a promising modality. Austen Riggs agreed to admit her on November 8, the day after her birthday.

Her father and I drove Ann to Stockbridge. She sat in the backseat, her legs curled under her, her head on the chest of the theatrical director, who made the three-hour trip with his arm around her. Unlike her relationship with Tim, this one seemed to be based on his need to care for her, and her need for his protection, rather than a passion or romance between them. Alex was polite but curt to her father and me. I think he saw us as the enemy.

I was struck by the beauty of the Austen Riggs Center. Two stately well-spaced white mansions were backed by the Berkshire foothills. No fence, no walls around them, the buildings looked like gorgeous private homes in the center of a charming village.

A nurse led Ann away. Her friend Alex left to visit friends he knew in the area. Bill and I had an intake conference with Dr. Jordan, the director of the institute.

Active childhood. Wonderful student. Goal-directed family. The story of how Bill, whose parents died before we finished high school, began his college education after our fourth child was born and finished with a master's degree from Columbia University. His writing. My work and writing. Ann's leadership with siblings and friends. Her own creativity—writer and producer of plays created to deal with social issues, actress in community theater. Her moving portrayal of Anne Frank. Advanced placement courses, Merit scholar. Her first romance the year we spent in Germany. Concern about her friends her senior year in high school. Africa. The unfinished thesis. The kindly silver-haired doctor had a prayerful way of touching his fingertips together as he led us through our memories.

No, he could not yet say how long Ann might need to be in residential treatment nor offer a more specific diagnosis than anxiety and depression.

Bill and I said good-bye to Ann in the hallway. It was hard for us to leave her. Brushing away tears with his clenched fists, her father went out to start the car. I walked through the stately foyer to the ladies' room, to wet two wads of paper towel and hold them to my eyes. I looked in the mirror and began to cry again. When the doorknob turned I fled into a toilet stall.

"Mom, are you in here?" Ann said. "I followed you down the hall. Oh, Mamma, you've been crying." She wrapped her arms around me.

"I'll be all right," I said, "I—I just want you to be all right again."

We stood in the little bathroom hugging, but her body was hard and tense against mine.

"Mamma," she spoke over my shoulder, "am I just being self-indulgent? Do you really think it's all right for me to take time out to be here? I know that other people must have the feelings I have but are strong enough to resist them."

"Annie." I pulled away from our embrace to be able to look at her face. Worry lines had creased her forehead. "What a terrible judge you carry around in that head of yours," I said. "This hospital only admits the kind of people who need it—people who can benefit from analysis. Be proud of your decision to come here."

Annie's eyes searched mine. "I'll be here a long time, Ma. The nurse said it takes at least a year to get better."

My heart sank. Although Dr. Jordan had been noncommittal, I expected Ann to be away about three months, the usual length of stay at psychiatric hospitals for patients I had dealt with. Had she made a mistake, opting for this analytic institute? Had Dr. Jordan assumed we knew that treatment here might take so long? I could not contain my tears, and Ann was crying, too.

"I followed you to cheer you up," she sniffed.

"Thanks a lot." I grinned, wiping my eyes.

" 'Bye, Ma." She turned left and was gone.

"Good luck, my Annie." I went out to the parking lot.

On the way home that night, Bill and I stopped at a small French restaurant. I told him what the nurse had said. Then my husband of twenty-three years told me for the first time that Ann's behavior had caused him to remember a long-buried incident. He too had fought an impulse to hurt himself when he was growing up. Recognizing some of the symptoms in Ann, he believed she could make a full recovery. His optimism lifted my own spirit.

Sharing a bottle of Chardonnay, we spoke about the time and money pressures that had come between us, and how long it had been since we had tried to share feelings. "I was trying to wait until you finished before addressing the distance I guess we both feel," I said. "I didn't want to add to your pressure."

The rest of the dinner and all the long drive home we talked hopefully about Ann, about what Richard might do when he finished college, about Billy's wish to go to Brown, and Ellen's ingenuity in caring for a horse in order to get to ride. We talked of the books we hoped to write, the trip we'd like to take if our money problems lessened.

Two weeks later, Ann's therapist asked that we attend a meeting with her. I went alone. Bill had to see his publisher.

Ann met me for lunch at the comfortable Old English Tap Room in the Red Lion Inn. She liked the program at Austen Riggs. The only requirement of patients was to keep four therapy sessions weekly and attend group meetings when scheduled. Ann spoke rapidly, but then we both did, and I ascribed the breathlessness to mutual nervousness and pleasure.

We wandered over to a small shop in the village center where Austen Riggs patients sold their artwork. I was alarmed when Jen, a barefoot girl with feverish eyes, told me she had been a patient at Austen Riggs for three years. "But not a single doctor has helped me as much as Ann has in the short time she has been here," Jen said.

In the waiting room outside the doctors' offices Ann and I sat opposite a young woman huddled in a velvet chair, her knees drawn to her chest.

"They're doing it again!" Suddenly the woman leaped from the chair screaming, "Goddamn it! Dr. Mills, where are you? Help me, Dr. Mills! *Help me! I need you!*"

Both therapists appeared in the waiting room at precisely two o'clock. The other woman threw herself at Dr. Mills. Ann kept her distance, following Dr. Feinberg.

The slim grave woman sat across from Ann with pen in hand. Ann bowed her head. The doctor waited.

"How long do you think Ann will need to stay here, Dr. Feinberg?" I finally asked.

"That will be up to Ann, Mrs. Craig. You may want to ask her yourself."

"Annie, do you have an answer?" I asked.

"I could tell you," Ann toyed with her fingers but did not raise her head, "what I think you need to hear, Mom. Of course I'll be out in time for spring semester."

"I do not *need* to hear anything, Ann, except that you are in a place which you are finding helpful."

I felt as though our forty-five minutes would be up before anyone said another word.

"Do you have a response to your mother, Ann?" the doctor finally asked. "Is Austen Riggs a place which you are finding helpful?"

After yet another silence, Ann said, "It's too soon to know yet."

When time was up, the doctor asked if I would come back monthly. I thought of the long round-trip drive. I would come if future meetings could be more productive.

Once outside, Ann spoke excitedly about her plans for our evening. "I want you to meet these wonderful musicians, Ma, called Stormin' Norman and Suzie. They're fabulous to dance to, and they're playing in West Stockbridge tonight. I went to hear them the first night I was up here."

"The first night you were here, Ann," I repeated, disbelieving. "All that night I couldn't sleep, worrying that you were feeling so alone."

"Well, you would have been right. That's why I decided to go out."

It seemed that the best table at the Square Rigger had been saved for Ann. The performers announced "a special song for someone we love" and blew a kiss toward Ann. A long-haired young man joined us. His eyes caressed my daughter. He introduced himself to me as the manager.

I drove home feeling angry and puzzled. While I was grieving that first night, she had gone out dancing. Perhaps I needed to see Dr. Robbins to address my own concerns.

Bill and I talked well into the night. I described the woman screaming for her doctor—how much sicker she appeared than Ann, yet how much more ready for help.

"Damn it, it doesn't make sense. I feel like we sent her off to some kind of posh vacation. Like the whole damn hospitalization is some kind of drama to get herself out of any responsibility for her paper or for growing up," Bill said.

"But think of Annie a few years back," I said. "The kid we used to know, who cared so much about her family and her future. I can't believe she would have chosen to avoid responsibility by being in a hospital."

"No," he buried his face in his hands. "Not in her right mind. She wouldn't. I just don't understand."

Later, I would find part of the answer:

> *Past:*
> *God this hurts*
> *Yippie yahoo to early school stuff*
> *so sincere.*
> *Sixteenth year*
> *surprisingly happy launching into love*
> *such sweet tenacious faith.*

Eleanor Craig

Violation.

Response: dichotomizing: bad/good
something awful happened/ help me!
Or no big deal/ I'm OK
so handle it alone. Grow up.

Of course, of course
I thought
refusing to be damaged.

Did I bury the pain
only later to be buried in it

I guess
I tried.

AUSTEN RIGGS, NOVEMBER 1975

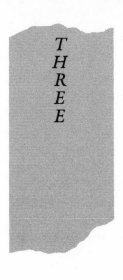

*T
H
R
E
E*

A Holiday
Without Annie

November 29 marked the end of Ann's third week at Austen Riggs. Our family made perfunctory preparations for Thanksgiving. But there was still a sense of holiday-on-hold until she could be with us.

Ellen put the cornucopia in the center of the dining-room table, taking care to have the fruits and nuts spilling from the basket, just as Ann always had. Then she put Ann's Pilgrim salt and pepper shakers and her silly cardboard turkey with expanding paper fantail around the cornucopia.

Ann knew how to do celebrations. Even in elementary school, she had seen to it that her birthdays had a theme, like her nautical party at seven or the ten-year-old birthday party when all the guests played detective.

All year long she collected costumes from thrift shops for Halloween. At one of her parties in Providence she dressed Mr. and Mrs. Carbone in heavy velvet robes, rescued from a defunct Shakespearean theater. With cardboard crowns, Ann pronounced them "King and Queen of the Eve of All Hallows." At Miss Cahill's whispered request, Ann draped her elderly neighbor in what had once been satin curtains and respectfully presented her as "Our Lady of Lourdes."

At home it was always Ann who led the kitchen songfest the night before Thanksgiving, while we made the stuffing and rolled out pie crusts.

Over the river and through the woods
to Grandmother's house we go. . . .

Before the traditional final song, "My Grandfather's Clock," Ann would rehearse her brothers to make the ticking sounds go ever more slowly, as she and Ellie stretched out the final words:

. . . but it stopped—short—never to go again
when—the—old—man—died.

The song always left me with a melancholy feeling.

This first Thanksgiving without her, we did not try to sing. Bill and I had had a serious argument over money. He took my concern as lack of confidence in his writing. I urged him to look for a job—college-level teaching—anything to bring a steady income.

"Like you do?" he said, referring to my modest paycheck. "Listen," he added. "I cannot write in an environment where I feel so unsupported. You are perfect. I am not. And I can no longer live with so much pressure."

After dinner he left the room to make a phone call. He arranged to have the use of a friend's New York apartment, at least until he finished his book. He left the house Thanksgiving evening.

I sat at the kitchen table looking at my manuscript. The only control I felt I could have concerning the future was for me to finish my own book. But that night, and many nights thereafter, I was unable to sustain the energy I needed to be able to write.

Flooded with ambivalent thoughts about my relationship with Bill, I put on a coat and went to sit on the porch. I felt pity for him. His own father had died on Thanksgiving Day, when he was just fifteen. His mother died the year we graduated from high school together.

We had accomplished so much since then. Bill entered college when Ellen, our fourth child, was born. By the time she was six, he had completed a master's degree and published an incredibly well-received book. I could understand his fear of trying to match that first success. He asked me to have faith. But I grew panicked as years passed and financial problems mounted, gradually broadening into issues of trust and control.

As a Catholic I had never entertained the thought of divorce. But I was ready to live alone rather than on someone else's terms any longer.

The phone rang at midnight of Thanksgiving night. I hoped that Bill was calling to talk. But it was Eileen Driscoll's mother.

There had been a terrible scene. Mr. Driscoll called his daughter a "whore" for appearing in the kitchen in her nightgown. Mrs. Driscoll read the note Eileen had written before she ran away. "I can't take it anymore," it read.

The police had been informed.

"I should have had the courage to leave," her mother said. "I would have spared my daughter."

Eileen was missing all weekend. Monday morning she was waiting on the steps at the clinic. I canceled my other appointments and took her out to breakfast. We spent the rest of the morning meeting with her parents.

Her mother wept. Her father glowered. I asked Eileen how she thought her parents would define the problem.

Eileen fixed her eyes on the floor. "My father would say, 'That girl is nothing but trouble.' My mother would say, 'Please don't do anything to upset him. You know how he gets when he's drinking.'"

"That does it," Mr. Driscoll got up. "I did not come here to get insulted by the one who's driven us crazy all weekend."

"See what you've done, Eileen?" Mrs. Driscoll sobbed.

"Are you going to leave without taking your turn?" I asked him.

"You heard her. The one who overdoses and runs away ends up blaming everybody else for her problems. Lissen, miss"—he pointed at his daughter—"I didn't have it as good as you when I was sixteen. You think I'm an alcoholic. My father beat my mother every night. There was no way I could control him. . . ."

In the process of telling his story, Mr. Driscoll returned to his chair.

Before the morning ended, we drew up a family contract that each person signed. I participated as a witness. Mr. Driscoll, having refused to consider AA, did agree to prove that he did not have a drinking problem by abstaining from alcohol for ninety days. Mrs. Driscoll promised that she would go to Al-Anon, not because of her husband, but to learn to manage her own life. Then she told about having been the childhood victim of an alcoholic mother who had died when she was just Eileen's age.

"Maybe," she mused, "that's why it's hard for me to relate to Eileen now."

Eileen's part stipulated that she would neither run away nor overdose. If she were to feel so helpless again she agreed to ask for an emergency family meeting.

Each person got a copy of the contract. We would meet every two weeks to check the family progress.

In mid-December I went to Stockbridge to visit Ann. We went to her bedroom to talk. She put on a tape of Bach's *Suite for Horns.* Sunlight streamed through the panel of lace she had tacked across the wide bay window. Ann had paisley shawls draped on each of three standing lamps. The window seat and both night tables flanking her bed were covered with antique toys I had never seen before—a metal bank with a dog that jumped through a hoop, little ladders with wooden acrobats, tin cars and trucks, dolls with porcelain faces, a Chinese-checker board with old glass marbles, kaleidoscopes, a gold candy box spilling with beads and trinkets.

"Annie, where did all this come from? How did you collect so much?"

"People here have yard sales every weekend, Ma. I didn't have to pay for most of it," she said defensively. "I always go at the end and lots of time they just give me all the stuff left over."

I sat on the window seat, she on the edge of her bed. I said it very succinctly. "Dad has moved into the city to finish his book."

"He's gone away to write before," she said.

"This time we had a fight before he left." I did not say that other times I had missed him and this time I felt relieved.

"I'm sorry, Mamma. I know it's so hard for you both."

Ann went over to her bureau. She tied a thin black ribbon around her head from which hung a large rhinestone star centering on her forehead, just above her eyebrows. With her eyes outlined in black, she looked like an exotic fortune-teller.

"Why the star?" I asked.

She glared. "I knew you wouldn't understand. It keeps me safe. That's all. I do not want to talk about it."

In the hall we met a thin young man.

"Mom, I want you to meet my friend."

"My name is Earthstar." He stared beyond me. "Earthstar," he continued, walking past us.

Again Ann was silent with her doctor.

"Is there more communication when I am not present?" I asked.

The doctor turned from me to my daughter. "Do you think so, Ann?"

"Sometimes."

"Ann," I said, "I'd think Dr. Feinberg should know that I told you about Dad and me."

"There's nothing to tell, Ma." Ann began to pick at her cuticles. "He'll be back when his book is done."

"I told you he had left, Ann, so that you could be somewhat prepared in case that is not true."

"It's too soon to know that, Ma. I don't want to talk about it."

Dr. Feinberg had been taking notes. She sat with her pen poised.

"Then let me bring up another subject," I said. "Do you feel that your time at Riggs is helping you?"

"It's too soon to know that, too, Ma."

"Why do you ask, Mrs. Craig?" the doctor finally spoke.

"I can't help questioning the value of Ann's being here to go to yard sales and nightclubs. And of my efforts to get here, only to participate in noncommunicative meetings."

"It must be Ann's decision how she uses her time," Dr. Feinberg said.

"Don't worry, Mom," Ann put her arm around my shoulder as we left the office. "I do feel as though I'm getting better here. It isn't easy for me to talk to Dr. Feinberg, but just being here is helpful."

"But Ann, it's important to tell your therapist if you are having a problem communicating with her."

"I have. I will again, Ma."

Ann declined my offer to take her to a restaurant. She raved about the candlelit dinners at Riggs. "You have to meet the cook, Ma."

John, in white apron and towering hat, was mincing pistachio nuts under a canopy of hanging pans. "My own version of a veal pâté," he said. He put down the knife and rinsed his palms before he took my hand in both of his. "Annie's mother! Oh what a pleasure, Mrs. Craig! I can't tell you what a wonderful girl you have here."

"Oh, sure you can, John. Go ahead and tell her!" Annie laughed.

"Honestly, Mrs. Craig," he continued to clasp my hand, "she's going to have to be a psychiatrist. When this girl started visiting me in the kitchen I began to tell her just a bit about my own life. I call her my own Dear Abby, don't I, Annie? She's done more than anyone else to help me see things clearly."

I left our family Christmas presents for Ann in her room. She packed up gifts she had made for the family—a writer's kit she asked me to send to her father, with a coffee mug and ashtray, a ceramic sugar bowl for me, small wooden boxes for each of her siblings on which she had shellacked collages. Richard's included Jimmy Hendrix and the Red Sox, Billy's a picture of Faulkner, Ann's rendition of the minibike he had once wanted, and a sketch of Tolkein's Middle Earth. Ellie's box had ballerinas and an actual photograph of Ellie jumping her favorite pony.

"I had no idea you could make these things," I said.

"You just don't get to see me in clay therapy," she laughed. "So give each person at home a big hug and kiss for me." She leaned into the car and kissed me good-bye again. "I hope that you and Dad will be okay."

I drove home with her gifts on the seat beside me, visible reminders of Ann's taking care of others, while remaining so closed off to receiving help for herself.

> Question:
>   What is the truth about needing others
> Thoughts:
>   I'm not sure
>   I think I feel that
>   Years ago I needed
>   in a way that was healthy
>   Then something odd about
>   over response
>   By others to me
> Somehow inappropriate
>   my simply human (I felt)
>   reaching out
>   Impact too powerful
>   not what I meant
>   always a surprise to me
> Question: Why?
> Answer:
>   Drugs, perhaps.
>   An easy explanation
>   Perhaps more subtle anguishes.
> Conclusion:
>   You learn not to hope for help
>   They are drawn to your strength
>   They would flee your pain
>
>   (DIARY ENTRY, DECEMBER 1975)

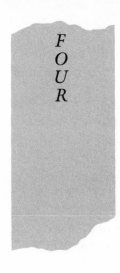

Suicide Watch

In February, Ann took a bus from Stockbridge to Danbury, for her first home visit. I was chilled by the sight of her stepping off the bus. Her smile looked forced, her cheeks white and sunken. She was dressed in layers of black: a black beret, long black scarf, flowing black coat, heavy black tights, and short black boots. She said she couldn't wait to get home. Her hug felt too intense.

Over the weekend, Ann spent hours in the kitchen making things she wanted Ellen and me to taste—tuna fish in heavy cream sauce, thick milk shakes, brownies loaded with peanut butter. We protested being force-fed, especially when she herself was not eating.

Saturday she shopped for a new pair of jeans. In the evening we saw a French film. Sunday morning she asked to be taken to brunch at the Café de la Plage, a waterfront restaurant, to celebrate some good news she'd been saving.

Lifting her glass she asked me to join in toasting the fact that she had been allowed to take an art history course at Williams College and had just attended her first weekly class. I wanted to believe it meant the beginning of her being able to pursue her old goals. But the pressure in her speech, the way she leaned too close, as if she had to persuade me she was better, made me apprehensive.

She kept the fork in her hand, but hardly lifted food to her mouth. She asked the waiter to pack up her meal. Her behavior in the restaurant, her obsessive preparation of food for others—foods with the soft texture of baby food—were all-too-familiar signs of danger. Her behavior made me fear that anorexia was becoming a strategy for Ann.

I thought about Stacey, a teenager I was seeing at the clinic. In weekly sessions, Stacey talked about her fear of losing control, and the effort to confirm the functioning of her mind by exerting control on her body by denying it nourishment. In meetings with her family, I supported Stacey's efforts to put her feelings into words, instead of waging war against her body.

On the ride home from the café I said, "Annie, I'd like to talk with you about your eating—"

"Please, Ma, stop. You are not my therapist."

"That's true, I'm not. I'm asking as your mother."

"And I'm answering as your daughter. That's something I will discuss with my therapist." After a pause she added, "Don't worry, please."

She spotted a tag sale, something we both enjoyed. I bought a lamp for three dollars. Ann knelt to search through cartons of used toys. She spoke to the young couple about remembered games of Twister and having had a Chatty Cathy doll like the one they were selling. They seemed charmed and urged her to take whatever she liked. Ann loaded the trunk of the car with boxes of games, a bag full of dolls and toys, and three cartons of books. I refused to let her take a mound of clothes that would not fit her.

Once home, she asked me to walk to the beach.

"I'd like to, but it's five o'clock. I need to get some work done so I can take the time to drive you to Stockbridge tomorrow. Ask Billy or Ellen."

She went to her room instead. At about one-twenty, startled by noises, I went downstairs and found her in the kitchen. No, she couldn't sleep, but she was "mighty hungry." Ann carried a tuna sandwich with a bowl of extra mayonnaise to her room.

At some point in my sleep I ground my teeth until I broke one. With an 8:00 A.M. emergency dental appointment and heavy traffic on Route 7, I pressed hard trying to get to Stockbridge in time to meet with Dr. Feinberg. Just across the state line into Massachusetts, I saw the state police car in the rearview mirror.

"Ma, listen," Ann said, as the burly policeman sauntered toward our car, "tell him you are speeding your crazy daughter to an institution."

The policeman stood with one hand on my window, the other on his hip.

"Officer," I said, "I'm rushing my daughter to a mental hospital in Stockbridge."

He leaned forward to look at Ann, whose fingers were flying in a kind of manic sign language. She smirked at him and began making cackling noises.

"Take it easy, lady," he said rolling his eyes, and backed away from the car. "Take it easy, now." He blew his whistle and held up traffic to wave us back on the road.

"You play crazy pretty good, kid."

"Slap me five," Ann laughed. The speeding incident seemed to have put us back in touch with the sense of togetherness we once had felt so often. As our hands connected she said, "You were right yesterday, Ma. Food *has* become an issue for me, but the freedom I have at Riggs makes it just the right environment for me to deal with the problem."

Her talking gave me hope of having a meaningful session with her therapist. I began to pick up speed again.

"Take it easy, lady," Ann mimicked the policeman. "Take it easy, now."

We were late. Dr. Feinberg had only a few minutes to spend with us. "How was your first home visit?" she asked.

"All right," Ann murmured, head bowed.

"That's all?" Dr. Feinberg jotted down a note.

"The one thing I really wanted to do with my mother," Ann said, "to walk on the beach, she was too busy to do."

"Ann, I can't believe that's all you have to say. We did all the other things you wanted. I told you I had to work in order to come here today. If you felt so deprived why didn't you tell me before?"

She bit her thumbnail. "I don't know, Ma."

Without comment Dr. Feinberg got up, indicating that our time was over. I felt angry at both of them.

"We had plenty of chance to talk in the car," I said to Ann. "Why didn't you tell me that in spite of all we did you hung on to the one missing piece?"

"I didn't realize it bothered me until she asked how the visit went," she replied.

When I got home, Ellen was upset. She had found a gallon of ice cream dripping all over the inside of the oven. "I feel angry at Ann," she said. "I felt like she controlled the house all weekend. I didn't even want to be in the kitchen when she was. And I really felt she was finding ways to keep you all for herself."

"Ann's got you running, Ma." Billy put down his guitar. "Ellie and I are okay. We don't need to compete for your attention. But don't you feel it, that no matter what you do, she isn't going to be satisfied?"

In spite of my belief in family therapy for others, I had overlooked the impact of Ann's hospitalization on my own children, or more specifically put their needs on hold in my mind to focus on the one I felt most needed my help. That night we had a family meeting.

Richard talked about wanting to join the Peace Corps after college. He choked up as he spoke about being worried about going overseas until the older sister he had been so close to was better. Billy was choosing a college. He wanted to go to Brown. I wondered whether Brown was really the best choice for him or whether it was his way of maintaining the deep connectedness he felt toward Ann. Ellen expressed fear that if her sister, who had always been her mentor, could become so unstable, perhaps it would also happen to her.

About two weeks after Ann had been home I found that she had left her black sweater in her room. It was covered with lint.

Readying it to wash, I found a pack of razor blades in the pocket. Terrified, I put in a call to Stockbridge.

"Dr. Feinberg, I have just discovered that Ann has been carrying razor blades."

"Yes?" she questioned as if to ask "So what?"

"Are patients allowed to walk around with razor blades?" I could not believe her casualness.

"How can we stop her, Mrs. Craig? If we were to take them away, Ann could buy another pack within minutes. The point is not her carrying them, but that she doesn't use them."

I did not hear from Ann or anyone at Riggs for weeks, until the night that Dr. Jordan called.

"I have to let you know that we have Ann on twenty-four-hour suicide watch. She is confined to the house, and someone will be with her round the clock. Nevertheless, we cannot guarantee her safety."

There had been a theft at the hospital. Ann was in no way involved. A full staff-patient meeting was called. Required attendance at the meeting meant that Ann could not go to the class she had begun at Williams College.

"Ann said, 'That does it' in a way that clearly indicated to us that she would be at risk if left unattended," the doctor continued. "I am sure you will want to come up but I would ask you not to do that. I will call you when we take her off preventive watch, unless there is reason to call before."

I called her father in New York. Bill was as shaken as I.

"Should we pull her out of there," he asked, "and put her in another kind of hospital?"

"I'm afraid to take the risk of interfering right now," I said.

Neither of us spoke for a moment.

"I guess we can't," he said. "She chose the kind of hospital she wanted. You can call me at any hour. I'm sorry not to be there with you."

As the evening wore on, minutes felt like hours and I was crazed by the waiting. I went into Ann's room. I prayed to my dead mother to watch over my daughter. At 9:00 P.M. I went to the car and headed up the thruway, not thinking of a destination. Around midnight I found myself on Charles Field Road, passing her old apartment.

At 6:00 A.M. I woke up at home on the living-room couch. Ann's baby picture and the soft stuffed monkey she played with as a toddler were on the floor beside me. I lay very still, aware of being upset by a dream, and trying to recall it.

Annie looked about ten years old. She had climbed to the peak of an enormous mound of gravel that had in fact existed at a construction site near our former home. Lots of other children, including Richard, Bill, and Ellen, were playing safely around the base of the pile. Ann called down from the top, "I am the king of the mountain!" She jumped and fell onto a ledge protruding half-way down the mountain. Picking herself up she swung her arms and crouched—in preparation for a second leap.

"No, Ann!" I screamed. "Don't do it! Let me come and help you."

"I am not afraid, Ma," she called and leaped into the air. Her body tumbled in slow motion. Her head was bleeding. She tried to get up.

"No, my baby! Lie still." I ran to her. "Just let yourself rest in peace now."

She lifted her head to smile at me, and then collapsed.

Dr. Jordan had my number at the clinic. I thought I would be better off if I went to work. I had been scheduled to present a summary of my work with Stacey to the staff. But as the therapist before me spoke about her own work with a self-destructive youth, I could not repress my tears and had to leave the meeting.

With Dr. Robbins I could only shake my head and weep. As words finally came, I kept repeating, "I don't understand. I just can't understand."

"I don't understand it, either," he nodded. "I felt I knew Ann well professionally and would never have predicted such a downward course in her illness. But even this crisis does not preclude recovery."

He asked if I had confidence in Dr. Jordan. I said I did trust the doctor. But confidence in myself had been shaken. How could I be so helpless with my own daughter and continue to work with other peoples' children?

"You have two sons and another daughter who are functioning well," he said. "As for you, personally, your ability to cope as well as you have, and to continue with your work and your writing, will all go to make you an even better therapist."

"I needed to hear that," I smiled weakly. Then I told him my dream.

"Your dream contained an important message," Dr. Robbins said. "There was no way you could stop her."

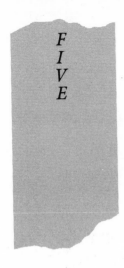

Waiting

The second night of waiting, Billy, Ellen, and I tried to talk about other subjects. But we kept returning to Ann. Billy thought each hour that passed meant she was less in danger. Ellen said she had prayed all day.

As the night wore on without a word from Dr. Jordan I became intensely anxious. I tried to write, to read, to watch TV. By midnight I found myself compelled to search through Ann's room. Somewhere I would find the clues, the information I could use to banish the imposter who had seized possession of my daughter's mind and body. Something in her room would help me to return to Austen Riggs empowered to release the funny, talented, hopeful Annie.

But the closets were jammed with black garments, the bureau packed with musty thrift shop bargains that told me nothing of the Annie I was seeking. The mounds of scarves, belts, pants, and blouses too large or too small to fit her, the baskets and battered velvet jewelry boxes spilling with rhinestone pins, bracelets, necklaces, bits of lace, single earrings, wooden beads a child might have strung, led me only to a sense of chaos—a feeling of utter helplessness. I got the plastic garbage bags, determined to rid her room of all the scrambled relics of other people's lives.

Annie, I am throwing away your toys the way you are throwing away your life. It is because I am so angry and so helpless that I have to do something—anything—connected with you, even if it is saying good-bye to things you have saved and touched. Beads and shells and stones and belts and shawls and books about food and handwriting analysis and religion, astrology, anthropology— pieces of you—like you are a piece of me—and you are throwing you away—and if you want to go and I cannot be with you—then I will *not* be left with these reminders.

I packed three bags and carried them out to the garbage shed. Her closet and bureau were still loaded. But my anger had been vented. I could stop now and allow myself to realize what I had learned: the sense of chaos and helplessness I had experienced delving into her belongings had to be what Ann felt also.

Early Saturday evening Dr. Jordan phoned to say the staff at Riggs felt Ann was no longer at risk. She would be allowed to return to her class at Williams College. In July she could resume home visits.

The Friday she came home was Awards Day for the children at the summer day camp I was running at our home. Richard, Bill, and Ellen were counselors. Billy rigged up his microphone and speakers for the ceremony. Richard played exciting drum rolls. Ann took on the role as master of ceremonies. I sensed a strain behind her dazzling smile, but even the most withdrawn child seemed delighted by her dramatic presentation of "the First Annual Camp Hopewell Awards."

The next day I was working at home when the phone rang. Eileen Driscoll sounded woozy. She said she had taken a bottle of Sominex and that she was sorry to disappoint me. She had gone home for a visit. Her father blamed her for the family problems. No, she was not alone. Her sister was there but did not know what she had done. Yes, she was willing to get her sister on the phone. Maureen agreed to keep Eileen moving. I called 911 and sped to the Driscoll home. In the ambulance, I held her head while she spat up the drugs. Eileen was admitted to the psychiatric unit.

* * *

Ann spent most of that day alone at Compo Beach, reading at her favorite spot, in front of the pavillion on the hard sand close to the water. She did not contact Alex, the theater director, or anyone at all. Sunday Ellen and I joined her, and we swam together between the jetties along the shoreline. Both nights I heard her in the kitchen after midnight. Her weight loss since she had been at Riggs was a nagging worry.

On Ann's twenty-fourth birthday, almost a year to the day she went to Austen Riggs, I received a call from John Sachs, who was both a friend and my insurance agent.

"Ann's medical insurance will only cover four more months," he said apologetically. "Aetna has already paid out almost fifty thousand dollars."

"I appreciate that, John," I said. I was grateful to Aetna for the coverage. But in the twelve months of her institutionalization, Ann's condition had worsened. I now had little hope of her getting well at Austen Riggs in the four remaining insurable months.

Families at the clinic had complained about it often—that discharge from private mental hospitals has nothing to do with the patient's mental wellness. It is fortunate if recovery should coincide with the length of insurance coverage. But treatment ends when money runs out, regardless of what the premature release of a patient may later cost society.

Two days after her birthday Ann called me to announce that she had been assigned to the one poor therapist for her situation. Her many friends agreed. Dr. Feinberg was all wrong for Ann. In an unprecedented move, the hospital allowed Ann to interview each of the doctors on the staff. She chose a young, bearded psychiatrist, Dr. Altbaum.

"I really like him, Mom," Annie sounded hopeful. "He wants to meet you too on November seventeenth."

The trees were turning late that fall. Driving up Route 7 was like gliding through a corridor of modern artwork.

I found Ann in her bedroom. I had not seen her since July. Her hair was sparse and lifeless, her lovely features lost in haunting hollowness. Her chest looked concave. With this much damage on the surface, what was going on inside her body?

She clung to me. I wrapped my arms around her. Her shoulder blades protruded sharply. "I, I—uh—made a terrible mistake, Ma," she said, each phrase beginning with a pause. "Dr. Altbaum is no better for me than Dr. Feinberg. In fact, he is really worse, and they won't let me choose again."

There was no point in leaving her at Riggs any longer. "Annie," I said firmly, "it's time for us to find a different kind of program. I want you in a hospital with a medical unit. I am very worried about your health. Your starving body is proof enough."

"No, Ma. I know what they do on medical units. I don't want to be force-fed."

We met with Dr. Altbaum. I said that I believed that Ann needed medical intervention right away.

The bearded, soft-spoken therapist would not support my position. "The choice must be Ann's alone. If medical treatment were forced against her will, Ann could pull the tubes and nothing would be gained."

I turned to my daughter. "Then let me take you to the emergency room at Northhampton Hospital and see if doctors there think you need to be admitted. I will accept their decision."

Ann stared right through me and shook her head.

"I cannot come back to see you, Ann, unless you agree to medical help," I said. "It is too painful, as your mother, to be asked to watch in silence while you decide whether to live or die."

At the door of the office building, I turned in tears to say goodbye to my wasted daughter. I was chilled to see her smiling.

> *What have I wrought?*
> *I would like to—*
> *I am desperately dying to*
> *Share my thoughts, my fears*
> *my self-contempt and pain*
>
> (DIARY ENTRY, NOVEMBER 1976)

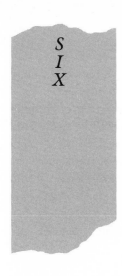

S
I
X

Leaving Riggs

Three weeks later Ann called, crying. "Mother, I am dying mentally and physically, and the mental part is the hardest." I remembered hearing almost the same words when Ann had called me from college.

I drove to Stockbridge through a blizzard. Her psychiatrist remained adamant that Ann should stay at Riggs and make her own decision there. But a nurse on Ann's unit said, "She can't go on much longer, Mrs. Craig. I have a feeling we touched her, but not enough to matter."

From a pay phone I called her father in New York. Bill and I were heading inexorably for divorce. He planned on relocating in the Virgin Islands, but I was glad he hadn't yet left. I needed his input about moving Ann. He too was frightened about her health and suggested that I call the Yale–New Haven Hospital.

Yes, they had one available bed in the Memorial Psychiatric unit. They might be able to admit her. They could do an intake late that very day.

I found Ann on her bed huddled under a blanket. "Who are you?" she looked at me vacantly. "I do not want you here."

"You're coming with me," I said. "You need a different kind of help now. You just rest and I will pack your things."

Ann tried to watch, but her eyes kept closing. As word spread that I was taking her, patients wandered in and out.

"I am Earthstar," said the strange young man who kept his eyes fixed beyond me, "who knows nothing of the ways and wherefores. But I will put my weight to the wheel."

The tall, thin young man continued to stare beyond me.

"Well, thanks." I tried to sound casual. "It would help if you could pack the books."

He turned mechanically and marched from the room. I did not expect to see him return. Two women began to help, but the task of packing became overwhelming as I began to realize the full extent of Ann's belongings.

I was deep in the back of Ann's closet when Earthstar returned with cartons and began to pack Ann's books.

The waiflike woman I had once seen screaming for her doctor entered barefoot and went directly to Ann, who hugged her close.

"Oh, Julie," Ann said, "I have to go. My family doesn't have enough money for me to stay here."

"I'll pack up your clothes," Julie said, shooting me a disparaging look and flinging Ann's strange collection of women's and children's clothing into one of Earthstar's cartons. She began to recite a litany of preferences. "I always liked boys better than girls." She folded a torn Persian lamb coat. "I liked my father better than my mother. I liked my uncle better than my aunt." Julie made trips from closet to carton with stacks of child-sized shirts and pants. "I like my brother better than my sister." On the closet shelf she found ten or twelve brown paper bags filled with withered flower arrangements Ann had received from friends and family. Julie began to pack them carefully.

"Ann won't need those." I shook my head.

"I want them." Ann glared at me.

"She wants them," Julie echoed. "I like my sister's father much better than my sister's mother."

Earthstar had packed only half a dozen of the hundreds of books when he stopped. "This must be systematic," he said. Finding a pad of paper he began to record each title, author, and publisher. In his wire-rimmed glasses he looked like a young professor deep into scholarly research. I wondered what his parents' hope for him had been.

Unable to hurry Earthstar, I decided to leave the books behind. Even with the capacity of my station wagon, I could see that Ann had far more than one load.

Elaine, a beautiful middle-aged patient whom Ann had introduced as "our New York Junior Leaguer," offered to help. She knelt in the closet to pack up the footwear—perhaps a hundred pairs of rubbers, boots, squared-off oxfords, gold and silver dance shoes, sneakers, most too large or too small for Ann.

I began carrying top-priority cartons out to my station wagon. The snow was already ankle-high and coming thick and fast. I wanted to get to Yale–New Haven Hospital by four.

My sense of urgency upset Earthstar. "Now, to start again," he said as he began to unpack the books.

Elaine gathered items on the window seat—glass bottles, dolls, old china cups and saucers. I felt I had an ally in her until she began to pack old food she found behind the curtains—little jars of jams and jellies, paper cups with mayonnaise and peanut butter, crackers, cookies, half-eaten sandwiches sealed in see-through plastic.

"No, Elaine," I said softly.

I thought Ann was sleeping but she leaped from her bed and placed herself between me and the window. Her eyes were full of anger. "I should not have let you come to my room."

"Ann, it isn't healthy to keep food this way."

"Go!" Ann pointed to the door. But she was weak, and moments later returned to her bed. The second time I said we had to hurry, Julie asked, "How much longer do we have?"

Earthstar studied his own bare wrist. "To infinity," he finally answered.

"Well, I cannot stand such pressure," Julie said and fled from the room.

I began to stuff the ratty fur coats, dead flowers, food, broken toys, and wrong-sized shoes into plastic bags.

"You can't be Ann's mother," Elaine shrieked, trailing me to the garbage bin. "Ann's mother would never throw her things away! I'll find out who you are. I'm going to call the FBI." High heels clicking, Elaine ran off.

Julie returned, her arms loaded with dead daisies, roses, lillies. She must have gone through the building gathering flowers, some clearly from wastebaskets.

"For you, Ann." She dumped the whole collection on the floor by Ann's bed, then waited anxiously.

"I like the flowers." Ann smiled.

"I like my mother's son better than my mother's daughter." Julie stepped closer.

Ann reached up from her pillow to touch Julie's hand.

"You are the only girl I ever liked, Ann." Julie sobbed and ran from the room.

My car was loaded, but three-fourths of the clothes, books, and toys had yet to be packed. Sharing my concern about the snowstorm, the kind nurse offered to put the rest in storage in the attic of the building. "You go ahead, Mrs. Craig."

Making one last check of things still left in her closet, I saw a stack of papers stashed in the furthest corner. Each of fifty or so pages was covered in tiny hand-printed notes, many with crossed-out corrections. Only the title page was neat.

Honor Thesis
Ann Craig
Brown University
May 1975

"Throw away?" the nurse extended a garbage bag.

I shook my head and shoved the papers in the bottom of my shoulder bag.

The nurse helped me put Ann's feet into boots, her icy hands into mittens. Over her black ragged coat we wrapped a soft pink blanket.

"I'll make another trip for the books," I said to Earthstar. I shook his flaccid hand. "Thank you for helping. I know you care about Ann. She's going to a different kind of hospital. She's going to feel better soon."

He moved slowly toward Ann. I waited apprehensively. Gently he ran his index finger straight from the center of her forehead, down her nose, across her lips, to her collarbone, then from her left shoulder across to her right. Earthstar had made the sign of the cross.

"Pray for all the souls of our departed," he murmured.

The nurse helped me guide Ann to the car. Earthstar followed us down the hallway to the outside door. All the way he whispered, "Good-bye, Moongirl. Moongirl, good-bye."

As I drove through the blinding snow, Ann made the bizarre hand signals we both had laughed about when I was caught for speeding and she wanted to show the policeman that she was my crazy daughter. But this time she could not stop herself.

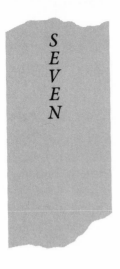

A Different Kind of Hospital

Ann had been at the Yale–New Haven Hospital for just three days when I met with the young resident on the psychiatric floor. "Your daughter is one of the most powerfully self-destructive persons I have ever encountered," he said.

"You make it sound deliberate," I responded.

"The sixty-four-thousand-dollar question," he smiled ruefully. "Does the patient choose the symptom? A question maybe God or Ann could answer. In any case we have to work out a plan for her here. I can't tell you how angry I feel, seeing that she was allowed to get into such god-awful shape."

"I hope that she can recover here," I said.

The doctor gazed at me. "Leave her alone awhile. See how she fares. We intend to set firm limits—weekly weight gain or feeding by tube. She's going to protest. We'll need your cooperation. As for hope? It's hard to say. It's really up to her now."

Ann called the following morning, crying into the phone. "Mamma, do you—you know . . . what they d-did to me?"

"What happened, Annie?"

"They—they said I had to drink this liquid meal called Ensure. They said I only had three minutes to do it. I told them I would, but I had to have more time. I said I hadn't been eating. They had to let me do it slowly. Oh, Mamma, you have to get me out of here. They're vicious," she sobbed.

"Tell me what happened, Annie."

"They—they pinned me down and stuck a tube up my nose. Oh, Mamma, it was awful. They poured the whole thing through the tube. Oh God, it hurt so. And now my nose is bleeding. Please, Mamma, come and get me."

"I can't come now, Annie. I cannot take you home until your condition is stable." I hung up the phone and broke into tears.

Ann bombarded me with examples of conditions at Yale. Unlike Riggs, where patients were trusted to come and go, Yale Memorial unit was locked. They looked ten floors down onto city streets. Getting out at all depended on one's status, weather, and the staff.

"We were scheduled for a walk today," Ann said. "It was drizzling lightly but that would have felt so good to us. Except the nurses didn't want to walk in the rain. So they herded us into the community room, put on a tape, and told us all to dance. Then they stood against the wall, making comments to each other about us."

"The freedom at Austen Riggs didn't make you better, Ann."

I remembered the bad joke: How many therapists does it take to change a light bulb? And the answer: One when the light bulb is ready.

In February, just two months later, when Ann's weight had climbed from eighty-two to one hundred, she was granted an afternoon pass. We decided to drive to the nearest beach for a picnic. She was still wearing black, but she draped a fringed blue shawl over her coat—a shawl that matched her eyes.

"I really have the eating under control now," she said as we rode the elevator from the tenth floor to the basement, which led out to the parking lot. "So much so that this place is debilitating for me now." She looked up at the hospital.

We stood in line at a delicatessen for take-out shrimp salad sandwiches. I saw two women staring. "Look how thin that girl is," one said, pointing.

I felt happy at the beach in spite of the chilly wind. We huddled together against the rocks. "Annie, it feels so good to be able to eat together again."

"I know, Ma. I needed Riggs as a time-out place. I got a lot from being there, and I'll always appreciate their philosophy. But as much as I've railed against Yale, being forced to eat has meant also being forced to let go of crazy magical thinking."

We both sat quietly for a while, watching the seagulls dive and soar.

"I have a funny animal story I never told you, Ma. It happened about three months after I got to Riggs. Late one night I was walking back from the Square Rigger when I found a porcupine by the side of the road." Ann paused to break off a piece of the butterscotch brownie we were sharing. "At first I thought it was dead, but it was only unconscious, so I called the Humane Society, the police, the dog warden. No one would come. 'Bring it to the nature center in the morning,' they said.

"I got a box and shovel from the greenhouse at Riggs. I made air holes in the carton, shoveled in the porcupine, and taped it closed. The porcupine never stirred, so I carried the heavy box back to my room and went to bed.

"In the middle of the night, the thing popped out like a monster. Suddenly it was strutting all around the room. I was a prisoner on my bed. I stood up holding my pillows in front of me while the porcupine circled, shaking quills all around the edges of my quilt. Then he toured my closet, loading the bottoms of my clothes with quills he was vibrating off. I escaped to the foyer and sat up all night on the couch. In the morning, John—you know, the cook—helped me catch him in the quilt and carry him out to the woods."

"Annie," I laughed, "submit that story to *Good Samaritan* magazine."

It got colder. The tide came in. We sat in the car in comfortable silence, watching waves break against the jagged rocks.

"I need to ask you something, Ann." I turned to her. "Why was food a symptom for you? I just don't understand. At our clinic I see people who had issues with food when they were growing up—food forced on them or withheld. But I really never thought of food as a problem in our house. Did you?"

I saw her turn away. Her foot began to tap. I waited through moments of silence. "Annie, why do you withdraw when I try to talk to you openly?"

She wouldn't look at me but she cupped her hand over mine. "It started in the hospital, Ma. I saw myself with no place to go. No school anymore. No life but the life connected to a mental hospital. And worst of all, I wasn't sure how much of a part I myself had played in making it happen.

"I looked at food—the one thing left that could make me feel good—that one last thing—just sitting down to eat—that still could make me happy. I had to take away that final pleasure. I did not deserve to have it."

"But why, Ann, why?"

"It was a prayer. Don't you see, Ma?" Her eyes pleaded with mine. "It was a final offering. A final thing to give up—as a kind of bargaining point to get me better."

Suddenly I thought of my mother and her transactions with God. My mother and food sacrifices: I'll give up eating all the treats I enjoy for a year, God, if only my husband, John, gets his deserved recognition. If my sister-in-law delivers her baby safely. If Eleanor recovers from the pneumonia. If . . .

"It was a prayer, Mother," my daughter was repeating. "Don't you understand? It was a prayer."

At the end of her third month at Yale, Ann weighed in at 110. Her body was gently rounded again, her hair shiny and bouncy, her face soft and beautiful. She was released to my care, and I was deeply grateful for her successful treatment.

We had a conference with her discharge planner. "We are all so pleased with the progress Ann has made here," she said. "Now we want her to find a job."

Ann reacted hesitantly. "I don't know what I could do."

I knew firsthand that work was a most powerful stabilizer. In the year and a half of separation from Bill, my life had focused on writing, visits to Ann, and work at the clinic. I had been appointed director of a day treatment program offering intensive therapy to young adolescents and their families. The work was so demanding that I had little energy to ruminate about myself.

In fact, I was at times inadvertently rude to friends—accepting invitations and finding myself unable to attend when the time came. Then Milton Fisher, a friend who taught a night school class on creativity, asked me to judge his adult students' projects. The invitation made me realize how isolated I had become. It seemed like an interesting event, and I accepted.

That night I met a publisher named Paul Green. "I think we could get creative about this ourselves," he grinned. "May I give you a call?"

Paul had four sons, one daughter, and Cookie, a cocker spaniel. I had two sons, two daughters, and Millie, a dog of dubious heritage. Our dogs sat in the backseat of Paul's car—Cookie behind Paul, Millie in back of me, staring out opposite windows, determined to ignore each other.

When we tried to blend our children, their first reactions were similar to Cookie's and Millie's. "Put nine kids together," Paul's youngest son Peter groaned. "If they made it into a television show I would never watch it."

Paul was kind and understanding. We both acknowledged sadness about divorce, the dissolution of the dream that our families would remain intact.

He offered Ann a job at his office. She began to learn graphics and layout and was at first faithful both to her work schedule and to keeping post-discharge appointments with the psychiatrist that Yale had recommended. But about three months after she came home, she started losing weight again, so drastically that her body soon looked as wretched as when she left Austen Riggs.

"It's so painful to see it all begin again," I told her.

"Yale made me put it on too quickly," she said. "It wasn't healthy to be forced to gain so fast. I have to do it my way." She began missing days at the job.

She did not like the psychiatrist Yale had recommended, and refused to continue to see him. She saw three other therapists, each one only briefly, insisting she was "therapied out."

* * *

Bill and I were divorced in March 1977. He said good-bye to our children and left to live in St. Croix, U.S. Virgin Islands, where he planned to continue to write.

Richard graduated from college and talked about joining the Peace Corps, which would take him overseas for the next two years. Billy left Brown for Boston University to work his way through college. Our family became fragmented. Ellen, still in high school, wanted to spend the summer studying art in Kentucky.

After her father left, Ann expressed concern about my deepening relationship with Paul. When he asked me to travel with him, she said, "Tell him you can only go if you have separate rooms, Ma. Say it's just too soon for any other arrangement. Let him know you're just not ready."

"But, Ann," I said, "what if I am?"

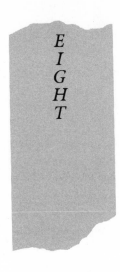

Getting Away

Paul was scheduled to participate in an international publisher's conference in Cairo. "I want you to come with me. But there is one condition: let's not bring our troubles with us."

I wondered whether I would burden Ellen, leaving her alone with Ann. But Ann had spiraled up again. She'd gained back some weight and returned to work in Paul's office. "Ann and I will be fine," Ellen insisted.

Still, the "old me" would have hesitated—if not for family reasons, because I felt too responsible to the adolescents in the day treatment program to leave for other than a scheduled vacation. But over time the pressures of my own life led me to heed advice I had often given to others: to take time for myself, time for personal renewal. Lately, this had meant simply an early morning walk or bike ride.

I would not turn down this chance to travel and to be with Paul. I raised my right hand and promised him a ten-day moratorium on all discussion about my daughter or his business.

The evening of the first vivid day in Cairo we sat through a sound and light show at the site of the Sphynx and the Great Pyramid. Deep amplified voices spoke the histories of ancient kings and queens and buried treasures. Lights played on the majestic structures. I pictured Ann's adventure—how she and Tim had climbed to the top of the Great Pyramid by grace of a full moon the night they had arrived in Egypt.

Too exhilarated to be tired, Paul and I taxied back downtown for a late-evening dinner organized by the publisher's association. All seven couples at our candlelit table joined in an excited exchange of first-day-in-Cairo stories. The thrill of the glamorous rooftop restaurant, the balmy starlit night, was heightened by sights and sounds on the chaotic streets below. Beeps from jammed-up cars and taxis entered a chorus with the hollow sounds of wooden wheels turning against cobblestone, braying donkeys, neighing horses, and whip-cracking drivers carrying wagons mounded with produce for the morning's market.

We rose as the president of the association offered a champagne toast to "What promises to be our most successful conference." Paul and I clinked glasses, nodding at our mutual pleasure in being together in this most dramatic setting.

"Ed and I don't usually come to conferences. We hate to leave our daughter," the woman from Texas began, as steaming broth was brought to the table. Her story stretched well into the lamb and vegetable dinner. Daughter Suzannah had almost finished college when one sadistic professor caused her to quit in protest. Jobs she took did not work out. Due to these misfortunes, Suzannah suffered depressions. Her parents paid for therapy.

Men at the table began to withdraw, tap fingertips, smoke cigarettes.

"Is your daughter manic depressive?" The gray-haired woman from Los Angeles sounded deeply involved.

"We never got a diagnosis. Suzannah's doctors would not talk to us, even in the hospital."

"I'm asking," the gray-haired woman said, "because that was my daughter's diagnosis, until we found out that her condition was entirely caused by sugar. Peg's behavior changed when she was five months old and started getting baby foods with sugar. By eliminating sugar from her diet, Peg is finally stabilizing."

"Most of the time," her husband said.

"Well, our daughter got to be too exhausted to work," one of the New York women said. "Then we heard about Epstein-Barr disease. A kind of chronic mononucleosis. There isn't any cure yet, but it helps to have a diagnosis."

"I never did hear about that Epstein-Barr," said a perky woman with a Southern accent. "But my daughter was exhausted also. She turned out to have low thyroid."

"Well," her husband cleared his throat, "taking thyroid has not completely cured her."

"She's improved a lot," the woman squeezed her husband's arm.

"Well, Suzannah's thirty-six and has yet to get a break. My own mother refuses to recognize that Suzannah cannot help herself. But Mother would never tolerate me having any problem either."

Suzannah's father downed another scotch and soda.

Mother/daughter relationships. At best, loving and empowering. At worst, toxic time bombs, ready to tick on in yet another generation of females.

My mother grew up with the uncertainty of having the father she adored disappear for days on yet another alcoholic bender. As a child, I could feel her episodic anxiety. I wanted to fix my mother's pain. I tried to cook and sew and make jokes to please her.

I always believed if my mother had only lived longer we would have come to the best of times. She would have loved her grandchildren freely, without the pressure of responsibility adding to her anxiety.

The push-pull of my relationship with Annie since her senior year in high school had become a gross magnification of the good times/bad times cycle I felt growing up.

"What's that you're humming?" Paul asked me on the elevator. I hadn't realized I was humming. The familiar song had taken on new meaning.

Rock-a-bye baby on the treetop.
When the wind blows the cradle will rock.
When the bough breaks the cradle will fall
And down will come baby, cradle, and all.

My own translation went:

When all is well between mother and her mother,
baby's life will be peaceful.
If mother's connection to her own family is broken,
the child will be the victim.

On the flight back to New York Paul took my hand. "It's hard to face reentry. We'll both be hit by the problems we tried to leave behind. But we aren't getting any younger. It's got to be our time, too. I don't want to wait."

We bought a dream house together—a cottage by the beach—and told our children that we were considering marriage. Ann and Ellen said they weren't surprised. They had discussed this possibility in our absence.

"We both like Paul a lot," Ann said, "and I appreciate the opportunities that he has given me. But don't you think you're moving rather quickly?" Paul's sons and daughter had the same reaction.

Marriage was harder for them to accept than divorce. It was more final. Each expressed happiness for us. But even young adult children have trouble letting go of the dream that someday their own parents might be reunited.

"You Craigs all love your father," Paul said at a family dinner. "I would not try to displace him. Nor would Eleanor try to be mother to Andrew, Alex, Douglas, Kathy, or Peter. You're all too old to take on another parent. I just hope we can all become friends."

In August 1978, surrounded by our children, relatives, and friends, Paul and I were married on the deck of our new home. Ann was the first to offer a toast.

* * *

On our combination wedding–business trip, Paul and I met my son Richard at a hotel in Seoul, Korea. Grinning broadly he said his own bride-to-be, Rosemary, was waiting in the lobby to meet us.

Two days later we followed the young couple from one government building to another. Rosemary and Richard's papers were scrutinized and stamped. "When will they be married?" Paul asked the man at the Bureau of Records.

"They just were," he said, handing a document to Richard.

The newlyweds were teaching English as a second language in distant villages. They would not be able to live together. I took a two-hour bus ride to see Richard's home—a single room with an outdoor pump for water—and to visit his class of fifty eleven- and twelve-year-old girls, all dressed in white blouses and navy-blue jumpers.

"Good after-morning, Mr. Mamma Craig," the official greeter curtsied. Richard let the children ask me questions.

A bright-eyed girl raised her hand. "Are you rich or poor?"

I paused a moment, thinking of their village, with neither electricity nor water. Yet all the children looked cared for, uniforms pressed, faces shining.

"I live in a pretty home right near the Atlantic Ocean," I said. "But most of all I have a good family and friends. They are what make me feel rich."

"Oh, very good. How-do-you-do." The questioner bowed.

I waved good-bye as fifty children stood to sing *Yellow Submarine*, the Beatle's song my son had taught them.

Richard walked me to the bus stop. The village sirens began to wail. People ran in all directions. He pulled me into a doorway. A formation of planes buzzed the area.

"A test," he yelled. "I hope," he added.

It was hard to say good-bye after that. With all the concern for Ann, I had tried to take for granted that my other three were safe and well. But September 1978 was a tense time to be in Korea. There were rumors of assassination attempts on President Park. Fearful of infiltrators from the North, the government imposed a curfew, which sounded at 10:00 P.M. Anyone out there-after was subject to arrest. I wished Richard could come home with me.

"Give my love to all the family," Richard said when the bus came. As I hugged him tightly he asked, "Is Annie really okay, Mom?"

"She seems much better, Rich. She goes out with old friends from high school. And Paul says she's got a natural talent for graphics. Try not to worry. I think she's really on her way now."

We flew back to New York filled with stories for the family. But the look on Ellen's face when she met us at the doorway stopped me.

"Something is awfully wrong with Ann," she said.

We raced up to her bedroom. Ann was grimacing, locked in pain with muscle spasms. Her legs curled backward underneath her body, her arms bent in against her chest. Paul carried her to the car.

She was admitted to the hospital with a 105-degree fever. No routine test revealed the source of infection. Finally, doctors questioned where and when she might have traveled. Ann told about severe bouts of gastrointestinal disorders she had suffered in Africa, information she had never shared with me.

The head of the department of infectious disease ordered more extensive lab work. "I am puzzled," he reported. "We know of no African disease that would explain her symptoms."

Thin again and depleted of energy, Ann was discharged. After three weeks of hospitalization, her record still read FUO—fever of unknown origin.

In the next six months at home, as her strength increased, she plunged into an enormous project—proposing to an editor/friend that she retrace the voyage of Marco Polo and write a book juxtaposing her own adventure with his. The editor asked for a twenty-page outline. Ann spent months collecting research.

I became apprehensive as stacks of books and notes piled up around her bedroom. Finally she allowed me to look through her proposal.

Setting the Scene: The Thirteenth Century
The dawn of the thirteenth century illuminated a continent
divided into squabbling realms. Nobility, monarchy, and church
vied for territorial dominance. Feudalism was at its height; the
lord in his stone manor reigned supreme. Peasants on his land
practiced stolid obedience, chained forever to the soil they tilled
but could never own . . .

The body of the book dramatically outlined the adventures of
the Polos and their return to their homeland twenty-four years
later, when all in Venice had assumed they were dead.

Ann wrote over one hundred pages but could not be persuaded
to show her efforts to the editor. "It isn't good enough. I need
more time to do it correctly. For now I'd like to move into the
city and try to find a job."

She asked for my support to help her sublet a studio apartment.
Having talked it over with Dr. Robbins, I decided to pay her full
rent for the first month, decreasing my contribution by ten percent a month so she could gradually assume the total responsibility.

Before she left, Ann stored the notes from her Marco Polo
project in the attic, close to the carton with her college honors
thesis.

She quickly found a job as a waitress for a splendid French
cook who had just opened a tiny place near Greenwich Village
called Evelyn's Kitchen. Paul and I had dinner there. A unique
crowd had found its way to the restaurant—off-duty police from
the local precinct station, gay young lovers, yuppies in blue blaz-
ers with gold buttons, venturesome middle-agers who had read
about Evelyn's "kitchen magic" in *New York* magazine.

From her easy banter, it was clear that Ann knew many of the
patrons well, especially Randy, a thin, hyperkinetic young man
whose eyes, like Ann's, were outlined in black. Randy came to
sit at our table, then made his way around the room.

A slim woman in a silk print dress introduced herself as Phoebe
Legere. "I love Ann so much," she said. "She is so beautiful, so
intelligent. I tell her she's got to get out of here and get a better

job. And she is always so encouraging to me in return. I am a musician. I'll be playing at the Rainbow Room in two weeks. Annie's spirit means so much to me. Your daughter is one in a million."

As Paul and I finished dinner, Ann's friend Randy was reading tarot cards for a policeman at the bar. The way she glanced at him while she worked led me to believe that Randy was someone special to Ann.

Her happy phone calls reporting how much she liked the acting classes she was taking between her shifts at the restaurant confirmed that Ann was thriving in her new environment. We tried to spend a day a month together. For me, having had little time in New York, our explorations were exciting. She led me up rickety stairways to tiny theaters in run-down buildings to see wonderfully talented actors in very far Off-Broadway productions and into small cafés where we could linger over cappuccino.

She began to talk about her future. "Ma, I don't know what it will be, but the more I look around the more certain I am that I have to find some new alternative for myself. For all that I love my family, we, like all families in our society, lack some method of communication—of supporting one another—the way I saw it in Africa. I saw whole societies there struggling with transition into modern times. I tried to understand their survival mechanisms.

"It must have been what I needed all along—what I hoped to find by going away—a survival mechanism. There were stresses pushing me I still do not have words for. I don't know how to do it, but I want to find some way of using theater to help bring people together. It's too much to face alone—the mega pressures of contemporary society."

"I don't know how you'll do it either, Ann. It sounds so overwhelming, to come to a city like New York and try to have some impact. But somehow it reminds me of when you were a little girl, and Dad and I used to watch you organize all the kids on Grove Point Road. You were the general even when the older kids were privates, remember? So I think it will take some time to figure out how to do what you want to do, but I bet you'll find some way to make it happen. Just be patient with yourself."

"That's encouraging, Ma," Ann said, putting her hand on mine. "Sometimes I feel as though I have to rush—to make up for the time I lost in the hospitals."

When her sublet ended, Ann called to say rents in the city had soared. She found a fifth-floor walk-up in an unimproved building on East Third Street. I was still naïve about the city. I told Ann about newspaper reports of runaways and drugs on the Lower East Side, but she insisted many people there lived quietly and securely.

I was impressed with the effort she made to fix her dingy apartment. Her paisley shawls now hung over the bathtub, which stood right next to the kitchen sink. She'd found a patchwork velvet quilt for her bed. Her Coptic art from Ethiopia was displayed across the wall above the wicker loveseat.

Heading out to lunch, we stopped at an apartment on the third floor. "Introducing Bobby!" Ann extended her arm toward the young man at the door. Bobby grinned and shook my hand. "Bobby and I are going to make it happen, Ma. Someday we're going to start a club together." Bobby nodded.

Passing the building to the right Ann said hello to the bag ladies sitting on the steps. Some she called by name. One in turn spoke her name.

"Isn't it sad, Ma? These women come here to Mercy House to be safe, but they're not allowed to bring their bags and wagons full of stuff inside, and they're too afraid that if they did go in to sleep, the things would be gone in the morning. So they sit all night on the doorsteps, guarding their possessions."

On my second trip to Ann's apartment, I found a long line of motley people—bag ladies, unshaven men, fur-coated matrons, men in three-piece suits—all heading slowly up the stairs into Mercy House. Annie called to me from somewhere in the middle of the procession. "We're on our way to pay respects to Sister Carmeline, the founding nun, who died in her sleep two nights ago," she said.

As we moved into the building, I saw within the open casket an ancient-looking nun, engulfed in black veil and habit. Suddenly a wild-eyed man ahead of us reached into the coffin and lifted the tiny corpse.

"Carmeline! Carmeline! Why? Why?" He kissed the nun squarely on the lips and lowered her head onto the white satin pillow. Then he pushed out through the crowd ranting "Why? Why? Why does it have to be—that the opposite of nothing is nothing. Why? Why does it have to be?"

The rosary from the nun's folded hands had caught onto his topcoat. The crazed man tossed the beads toward the casket. A priest caught them.

"Excellent save, Father," someone murmured. "Excellent."

Ann paused outside to talk to a woman rocking a shopping cart piled high with papers and rags. "How are you, Sophie?"

The woman's lips tightened. She looked ready to strike. Her hand shook as she pointed to my daughter. I hoped that Ann would leave, aware that she had trespassed. But the woman's voice was gentle. "Annie, Annie."

"Sophie, remember I told you that someday you'd meet my mother? Well, here she is." Ann turned to me. "She came down from Connecticut to see me."

To me Ann whispered, "Mom, got a buck or two for Sophie? I'll pay you later, honest."

I gave Sophie three dollars. She tucked the money down her shirt, then drew a dirty rag out through the side of her shopping cart and pressed it into my hand. I did not want to touch it. But there was no refusing.

"Wait, Ann." Sophie dug through the mass of clothes and papers, working her way to the bottom. "See, Annie, see." The toothless woman pulled out a sooty envelope from which she took a frayed and faded picture of a sweet-faced woman holding a chubby infant. "I had a mother. I also had a mother."

"She was beautiful, Sophie."

Sophie pressed the picture to her lips, then tenderly slid it back into the envelope and returned the proof of her own identity to its place underneath the layers of other people's discards. Without a good-bye, Sophie pushed her cart across the busy street.

We watched her turn the corner before I went to the refuse container to deposit Sophie's gift.

"Uh-uh, Ma." Annie's hand restrained me. "Sophie's territory goes anywhere from here to Grand Central Station. In fact, I've seen her checking trash bins in the station. She would know you didn't like it if she found it. That would really hurt her feelings."

On the train ride home I wondered what Sophie's mother had envisioned for her baby. Had she borne another child, who lived a different life-style?

I thought of my dreams for Annie. Early on, that she fulfill her own wish to become an anthropologist. That she would know the joy of having children. Later simply that she would survive. And now, that she would find her life rewarding, however different from what I had once envisioned for my firstborn.

Before I went to bed I scrubbed Sophie's scarf in the bathroom sink and ironed it on a towel. Then I tried it up against my pink sweater. It was rather pretty.

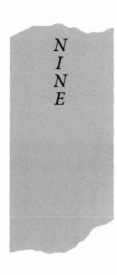

The Fashion Show

The sound of the phone at midnight woke me with a start. I reached for it, fearing someone in the family was sick or a client might be in trouble. But it was Ann calling from Evelyn's Kitchen.

"Sorry to call so late, Ma, but I had to tell you. This top European designer just had dinner here. He said he loved my makeup and that he was short one model for his show tomorrow afternoon. He asked me to be in it! It's at two-thirty at a fancy club called Xenon on Forty-seventh Street. Any chance you could come to see me?"

I hesitated, trying to remember whose appointments I would have to reschedule. But the more powerful thought of all the trips I took to see Ann in unhappy circumstances made me answer unconditionally. I owed myself a chance to enjoy her achievement.

I could hardly believe the size of the crowd. People were jammed shoulder to shoulder from the doors of the disco all the way across the street. The mob was wild and growing. The entire block had been cordoned off, patrolled on both sides by a line of mounted police. I tried to make my way to the closest of the many doors, pushing past a young man wearing ruby-colored earrings the size of golf balls, a fat man in an ermine coat, women wearing tafetta gowns, and a group whose sex I could not determine, dressed from head to toe in gilded leather.

Suddenly a frenetic young man in an ankle-length tweed coat and gray fedora caught me by the wrist and led me through the throng to a side door of the theater. "Remember me? I'm Ann's friend. Randy Slade," he called back over his shoulder. "Annie wants to see you.

"Wait here." Randy left me by the door.

My excitement grew as I waited. Perhaps Annie too compared this happening to all the hard times we had been through and wanted to share this moment of pleasure.

When the thick metal door finally opened a crack, it was too dark inside to tell who was there until I heard her voice.

"Go home, Ma," she said flatly. "I have changed my mind. I do not want you here."

I felt totally bewildered. "Annie, something must have happened. Why would you change your mind when I've come all this way to see you?"

"They won't let me do my makeup. They won't let me fix my eyes. The way they have done it to me, my face looks fat and ugly."

Even in the shadow I could see the outline of her cheekbones. "Oh Annie, that's crazy! You are so far from being fat—"

"That does it!" She began to shut the door. "You came all this way just so you could tell me I am crazy."

"I can't believe you could be so unfair, Ann. You told me to go home before I said a word. Don't twist my words to push me away."

"Then do what you want." She closed the door. There was no handle on my side.

I didn't know what to do. If this were simply stage fright and she could pull it together I wanted to be there to see her. The whole row of doors at the front of the theater swung open simultaneously. Suddenly I was caught in the forward surge of the raucous crowd. We moved through a lobby into a hall with purple velvet walls, scarlet velvet chairs, flashing strobe lights. I found a side chair with a good view of the stage.

"One look at your face and I said to myself, 'Get that lady a vodka.' " Randy reached over my shoulder to hand me a glass.

"My guess is that Princess Annie disinvited you like she did the rest of us."

It helped to hear that I was not the only person Ann had tried to dismiss.

"That gal's just got the jitters." Randy settled momentarily in a chair behind me. But he seemed nervous also, and kept leaning forward, tapping my shoulder.

"Your daughter is a shooting star, Eleanor. I can tell she's going to make it big in New York. She has lots of fans already. She's like a guiding light to all of us."

The theater darkened. Spotlights swirled around a seminaked black man in a silver loin cloth, beating rhythms on a ring of conga drums. The lights expanded to illuminate three other musicians, and then the strobe lights focused on a line of models strutting back and forth on the T-shaped runway.

Somehow, as models flashed open jackets to show revealing tops, twisted and twirled to display wide-splitted skirts, I thought about the fashion shows at Our Lady of Mercy parish house. Father Mealy would have called for a perfect act of contrition, not just from the models but from every Catholic watching.

"*Bienvenidos, amigos!*" the drummer shouted. "*Vamanos a una boda española!*"

The grand finale—a Spanish wedding. Ann would have to be in this scene, unless she left without performing. First the bride in a short strapless dress congoed out. Then her gaudy attendants each in different shades of Day-Glo color. Wedding guests arrived to dance around the bride and bridesmaids. The audience rose, swaying to the pulsing drums.

I stood on tiptoe searching for Annie and finally caught sight of her briefly—the only person walking through her steps, almost numbly, in the string of models snaking ever tighter around the bride. At the final earsplitting drumroll I saw Annie flee from the stage.

Behind me, Randy murmured, "Ohh-ohh." I turned around but he was gone as well.

I was among the first to get to the stage door. After several minutes, the models and musicians began coming out, to be greeted by waiting friends. But Ann was not among them. When the final cluster dispersed, the police began removing the cordons. A man in jeans came to close the door. "Don't know who you're waiting for, lady, but I'm the only one left."

I raced up the street to look for Ann. I searched in all directions at the crossroad, then went into Nathan's restaurant on the corner, hoping she had stopped for coffee or even just to hide there. I looked in Nathan's ladies' room, and then in stores and coffee shops all the way down Forty-seventh Street.

Finally—angry, disappointed, sad for Annie, and sad for myself as well—I gave up and walked back to the station.

At home there was a message on the telephone answering machine. Her voice sounded hoarse.

"Ma? This is Ann. I didn't mean to worry you. I just had to be alone, that's all. I'm okay now. Thanks for coming in. Someday I'll make you proud of me. Love you very much, Ma."

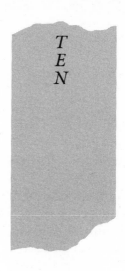

The Pyramid Club

Ann came home to tell us she and her friend Bobby had found a usable space where they might turn their dream to reality. In a vast empty storage area behind a dingy bar on Avenue A they would open a new kind of club—a coming-together place where unknown performers, new bands, and avant garde filmmakers would exhibit their talents.

Ann's version of the club-to-be had yet another dimension: "I see it as an opportunity, Ma, a precious chance for better communication. There are so many social conflicts here—the poor being evicted to make way for co-ops, drugs being pushed at powerless people to keep them disenfranchised. We're going to put on shows that offer clarity and hope to people from the East Village to Wall Street. If we can unveil the differences, and help each other find some commonality, and do all that with humor, maybe we can be a tool for change, offering a sense of what we all might become if we could work together. I hope this isn't sounding too pretentious, but I keep thinking of what Armstrong said before they lifted off from the moon. Remember how we watched together in that little café in Europe?"

"Sure, I remember." I smiled.

"I think the words were something like 'Here men from planet

Earth first set foot on the moon.' " Ann stared out the window at the evening sky and then spoke very slowly. "We came in peace for all mankind."

To Paul she spoke about a club that would "search for fundamental patterns," where she herself might have a voice "in intergrating a wide range of individuals to a sense of collective awareness."

Six months from its conception, the Pyramid Club opened to the widely divergent audience Ann and Bobby hoped to attract. Wall Streeters in three-piece suits soon waited with transvestites, people with rainbow hair, well-known performers, political activists, and long lines of voyeurs. *The New York Times* wrote it up as a new "in" place to be seen—the cutting edge of entertainment for 1983. Ethyl Eichelberger, a rising performance artist, described Ann in the *Village Voice* as "the best M.C. in New York."

The first time Paul and I headed for Avenue A to see Ann perform, the taxi driver refused to take us. "You folks don't want to go down there. It's dangerous," he said.

The line in front of the Pyramid Club stretched a block and then around the corner. By identifying ourselves as Ann Craig's parents to a doorman with an Apache haircut and leather jumpsuit opened to the waist, we were spared the wait. We forced our way through the crowded bar to one of the tiny tables that ringed the dance floor. Ann was already onstage. Wrapped in a black sari, with a black lace skirt as a mantilla, she held the audience enthralled as she danced to a pulsing drumbeat.

The music stopped. "The promised moment has arrived, folks!" Ann announced. "It's time to welcome six extraordinary debutantes, whose very presence with us tonight represents six incredible victories of triumph over adversity. For tonight, folks, for the first time in their lives, each of these debutantes is ready to reveal to us the most intimate, most devastating experience she has suffered as a result of being here in New York. And we ask you to listen carefully to each compelling sociological and historical dialectic, for before this night is over, you—yes, I do mean *you*—will choose the winner of the first Annual Vicky Award!"

Ann worked the stage with the microphone, one section at a

time, gathering in the crowd with her mesmerizing eyes and hypnotically paced delivery.

"Ah, yes! I hear you. I can hear your murmurs. And what, you ask, is the significance of this first annual award? Tonight, my friends, we need your clarity and concentration. Brace yourself to hear the stories of our six lovely victims. Then you will be asked to decide which one among them has been the greatest victim in the city of New York. And we will crown that person. Yes, crown her here tonight. Miss Vicky 1983!"

The crowd roared with enthusiasm. To a wild drumbeat, the curtain behind Ann rose, revealing five members of a pulsating rock band: Each musician dressed entirely in black; each had a different color of hair, including buttercup yellow, cherry red, and Kool-Aid grape. Ann danced onstage alone for several minutes, then held up her hand for the band to stop.

"Patty is ready now, folks!" Ann gestured to her left, as a tall gorgeous redhead, lushly molded in a strapless silver gown, gracefully approached her. Ann adjusted the microphone stand up, as Patty, twisting a lace handkerchief, launched into a woeful tale of being mugged on her thirtieth birthday.

"She's beautiful," I whispered to Paul.

"She's a he," he answered.

"No!"

"Yes!"

"Thank you, Patty." Ann patted the speaker's shoulder comfortingly. "Thanks for sharing such a difficult story. We're all wishing you a much happier birthday next year. And now folks, meet Lucinda!"

An even more sultry, delicate-featured blonde in a pink ball gown came center stage from the right. "Lucinda," Ann nodded sympathetically, "our handicapped debutante! Yes, friends, until the age of three Lucinda was a happy, healthy little creature. Then tragedy struck. Lucinda suddenly sprouted, not one, but two extra personalities! But Lucinda herself will tell the rest."

Eyes darting furtively, Lucinda trembled. "I—I liked my three personalities. Ever since I was three, I had someone else to play with. And—and then last year I came to New York, from Omaha,

Nebraska, because one of me always wanted to be a dancer at Radio City Music Hall. But instead they sent me to—oh, Ann, I can't go on—" With a tragic expression, she turned to Ann.

"Shh, it's all right." Ann grasped Lucinda's hands, "We'll wait until you're ready." The audience hushed.

"They—they put me into Bellevue for psychiatric observation. They—they said what I had was wrong. People aren't supposed to have three minds in just a single body. And then they," she sobbed, "they made my two other friends go away. If I hadn't come to New York City, I could still be Siamese triplets!"

The crowd roared with laughter.

"She's really funny," I said, clapping.

"*He*," Paul answered.

Four more stunning-looking transvestites recited. All six remained onstage, as Ann reviewed each story, one by one holding up each victim's hands like the referee at the end of a boxing match, each time evoking thunderous audience response. The crowd clapped and cheered their "vote" for Miss Vicky.

"Yes, you did it! Thank you, folks! According to my Applause-o-meter," Ann checked her watch, "our winner tonight is Melissa (cheers), who you obviously agree suffered the most harrowing experience of all. Yes, folks, it was our own poor Melissa who went back to visit in Bronxville and—and—it's hard to repeat it—*got along with her parents!* Melissa—" Melissa bent, and Ann crowned her with a papier-mâché replica of the Statue of Liberty's headdress, only this one glowed with tiny Christmas lights. "Let's hear it, folks! Melissa! The victim of the year. We now pronounce you Miss Vicky, 1983!"

"Ann is incredible!" Paul yelled in my ear above the cheering crowd.

"The kid I was so worried about," I yelled back, "is making her dream a reality."

Paul grabbed my hand and squeezed it. "I worried, too. Don't you forget that."

I nodded and blew a kiss to him.

Miss Vicky blew kisses to the audience. The doorman who admitted us delivered a note onstage to Ann. To read it, she shielded her eyes from the arc of spotlights. Again Ann stopped the band with a gesture.

"Wait, folks—just hold on a moment! You're never going to believe it! Ladies and gentlemen, you are privileged tonight to witness a first in all the history of our wonderful Pyramid Club. Tonight, for the first time ever, we have in our audience (long pause) *genuine parents!*" As the audience clapped and roared, Paul and I were suddenly caught in flashing strobe lights.

"And they're *my* parents!" Ann's magnified voice blared out, increasing the wild response as Paul and I, blinded by the brilliant lights, rose to wave and bow.

We had arrived at eleven. At 2:00 A.M., Ann left the stage to tremendous applause. Suddenly, Ann's friend Randy appeared to Paul's left. "Isn't she absolutely fabulous?" he shouted over the blaring music. "Follow me, I'll take you down to the dressing room."

Paul and I struggled to trace Randy's erratic course through packed-in dancers to a side door that led to a dark narrow stairway. "There's a miniclub down here," Randy said.

It took a moment to see. Randy had to be joking. The darkened cellar seemed only to be a storage place for stage props. Giant set designs rested against walls. Like a fantasy forest, papier-mâché palm trees, gaudy totem poles, and six-foot-tall cardboard candy canes sprang from concrete floor up to the maze of silvery pipes overhead. Crouching, we followed Randy through a tunnel created between a leaning stage set and the left side wall. We came out to a candlelit bar, flanked by two shabby couches. Ann, surrounded by a group of men, sat on a high stool at the bar.

"Randy," she glared at him. "I can't believe you brought my mother here." A young man dropped a cigarette, ground it into the floor and kicked the remains under the bar. He and several others walked away.

"Well, welcome to our inner sanctum," she held out her arms to Paul and me. "My friends here were being naughty tonight—smoking a funny kind of cigarette—and I was just telling them not to. Then I was going upstairs to find you."

"Ma, Paul, meet Masao." Ann turned to a Japanese man. "And Gunther and Wilhelm, who are both from Frankfurt, Germany."

The young men rose to shake our hands. "Your daughter vas great tonight." Gunther nodded seriously.

"And Tron." Ann turned to the only person at the bar. "You have to meet my parents."

The tall slender person unfolded himself from the high stool. Without the tumult of artificial curls, and with only traces of lipstick, rouge, and eye liner, Tron still wore the shapely dress that made him instantly recognizable as Miss Vicky.

"Congratulations on your award." Paul grinned.

The young man's gentle eyes turned to Ann. "Your daughter's the one who deserves the awards," he said softly. "She inspires the best from each of us."

"Here, here," a trio from one of the couches raised their glasses in salute to Annie.

"Oh no!" Ann clasped her hands against her chest, feigning embarrassment. "Thank you." She curtsied. "Thank you all." She blew kisses.

"Okay, Miss Universe, awards night continues at the Pymander Delicatessen," Tron said.

"Mamma, we need a few minutes to change. But Paul—just you wait. Wait till you taste those sour cream blintzes!"

Ann and Tron disappeared. Paul and I waited twenty, twenty-five, thirty minutes. Randy and the others went upstairs. Our calls to Ann went unanswered. I was reminded of looking for her after the fashion show at Xenon.

"Maybe there's another exit and she expected us to meet her elsewhere," Paul said.

"No," I said. "I think she was angry about Randy bringing us down here."

"I think that was because of the pot." Paul stopped talking. Tron and Ann reappeared, he in boots, jeans, and a tight black sweatshirt, Ann in a black shawl and dress with above-the-knee hemline cut like rose petals.

"Mother?" She seemed surprised to see me.

"Are you okay, Annie?"

"We're fine. Fine." Tron put his hand under Ann's elbow and led us all toward the stairway. "Sorry to keep you waiting. We got to critiquing the show and lost track of time."

Over wonderful blintzes, Ann asked about Richard's new job in Washington, D.C., the news from Billy and his fiancée, Nicola, who had joined my former husband in St. Croix, and how Ellie's artwork was going at college.

When she got up to find the rest room I followed her and leaned against the sink in the tiny space. "Annie, you were great onstage. So funny and natural. And you look beautiful. But the scene downstairs disturbs me. If working there means involvement with drugs, it isn't worth it, Annie. You've been through too much to take that kind of risk with your mind and with your body."

Ann lit a clove cigarette and turned away to blow out the heavily scented smoke. "I was afraid you'd think that, Ma. It's not the scene at all. Sometimes people bring a little pot in, like those German boys tonight. And I might take a drag to take the edge off. It's so hard to go home and sleep after getting so revved up to do a show. Don't worry, Ma." She doused the cigarette under the faucet and flipped it in the waste container. "I know what I'm doing." Ann hugged me.

"Sure, I think they lost track of the time because they'd been smoking pot," Paul said in the cab. "But they certainly sounded fine at the restaurant."

Paul and I, who were usually asleep by eleven, had to ring for the doorman at the Princeton Club. "Can you believe it—us being out till four-thirty!" he said. "Well, life-style is bound to change for the parents of a star."

On October 15, 1983, Ellen married her high school sweetheart, Charlie Perlwitz. She chose her sister Ann and Richard's wife, Rosemary, to be her attendants. Ellie and Charlie were radiantly happy. Ann looked thin and shaky. As she stood at the altar next to her sister, her shawl slipped, revealing her frighteningly bony shoulders.

We had the reception on our lawn, by the saltwater pond.

"It was the bravest thing I've ever seen," a friend said to me, "for Ellen to let poor Annie be her maid of honor."

"Ellen wouldn't have it any other way," I said.

On Thanksgiving Eve, Ellen and Charlie went to see Ann perform. Charlie—a conservatively dressed broker—got hugged by the doorman, dressed in wedding gown and veil.

Ellen raved about the show, written and directed by Ann, who also read the part of Squanto, the Indian Brave. . . .

> *Yes, they parked on a rock*
> *and they disembarked*
> *Funny looking creatures all white and stark.*
> *Took over our land without asking please*
> *Built funny houses chopped down our trees*
> *always talkin and braggin about being free*
> *But those folks gobbled land*
> *From my people and me. . . .*

At scene's end, Indians and Pilgrims, linked arm in arm, chanted:

> *No more acting like turkeys*
> *No more gobbling in greed*
> *Freed to help one another*
> *Brothers—sisters in need*
> *These are harvest years friend,*
> *You will reap what you sow*
> *Reach with hearts opened fully*
> *As we did long ago.*
> *Happy Thanksgiving!!!!*

Scene Two switched focus to the gentrification of the Lower East Side, the displacement of the poor and minority peoples, and ended with a repetition of the final verse the Indians and Pilgrims had recited.

"Ann was great, Mom. Funny, and at the same time conveying

a message. But after the show we went out to a delicatessen together. She was talking too fast. Her whole body seemed jumpy. Charlie thought she might be speeding. I'm sorry to tell you, but I know you'd want to know."

PYRAMID

I had the chance to step
into a hedonic yet potent
world and speak.
It was a creepy other-defined world
I was tackling
but worth attempting.
Reach them
and they define so many others.
And I had the chance
but I succumbed
publicly and
invisibly
and invalidated every message
I was trying to convey.

(NOTEBOOK ENTRY, 1984)

Heroin

During Ellen's three-day break from her studies at SUNY Purchase, she and I made plans to meet Ann for lunch at the Cupping Room on Broome Street. We waited from twelve to one. Then we ordered without her.

The waiter was leaving the check when she finally appeared with Randy Slade. Sitting opposite me, Ann began to peel off layers of black sweaters, a shawl, a scarf, under which she wore a long black T-shirt over skintight leggings.

Randy never did take off his wide-brimmed gray fedora and ankle-length tweed topcoat. With manic gestures, he spoke of trouble he and Ann had finding someone they just *had* to meet before they were able to join us. Ann picked her nails and occasionally looked from Randy to me. Our eyes met and she tried to smile.

Randy ordered two cappuccinos with Kahlúa. He spread out an astrology chart and began a dialogue with Ann about ascending planets as if they were alone. She paused to sip her cappuccino. Her head began to nod and she almost spilled the drink. She caught herself and sat up straighter.

"Are you okay, Ann?" Ellie put her hand on her sister's arm and looked at me in alarm.

"Juss-tired-Ella-bella." Her words slurred.

"You scared me," Ellen said.

"Honest," Randy waved his arms, "if you two saw how much energy this girl put out on the stage last night you'd say it's a miracle that she even got up today."

"I do know how hard and how late you work, Ann," I said. "But something else is going on."

"What are you saying, Mother?" Ann leaned toward me until her nose was inches from mine. "You think I'm nodding off on drugs, is that it?" She glared at me.

"I don't know. If you were, I'd want to help—"

"That does it!" Ann scooped up her scarves and sweaters and stormed out of the restaurant. She dashed across Broome Street and disappeared around a corner.

"That's all for now, folks." Randy rolled up the astrology chart and with it waved good-bye.

I described the meeting to Dr. Robbins.

"I've been working with a fine young therapist," Dr. Robbins said. "His name is Norman Itkowitz. I think he could help you. He is clinical supervisor at Liberation Clinic in Stamford. I have a lot of respect for the support they offer family members when drug use is the problem."

I wasn't ready to call Liberation Clinic. Their program was designed to offer methadone for heroin addicts. I would not let myself believe that Annie could be in that kind of trouble.

"The number you have called is no longer in service." I dialed again to be certain I could not reach her by phone. Then I went back to New York to find her. I banged on the door of her apartment, waited in the stench-filled hallway, and finally left a note: "Please call me, Annie. I am looking for you. Mom."

The bartender at the Pyramid Club said she hadn't done a show for weeks. "A guy called Randy came in to say she'd gone away."

March and April passed without a word from Annie. Arthritis pain I had not felt since the time of my divorce returned to plague my hands and joints. At the end of a session Dr. Robbins asked me how I could take care of myself, in spite of the waiting and hoping.

The answer did not occur to me at the moment. But later that day I decided that the best thing I could do for myself was to get on with my writing. My third book, *If We Could Hear the Grass Grow*, about the therapeutic summer camp my children helped me start, was published in 1983.

Although I had a contract for the book, I felt I had lost my ability to write. To try again, I had to get away from all distraction. I applied for and received a three-week fellowship at Cummington Community for the Arts, in Cummington, Massachusetts.

Paul joked that when he traveled it was business, but when I had to go it felt to him like desertion. I knew that behind the comment he was feeling pressured by uncertainties in his own work, and that it would be hard for him to be alone. But he helped me pack the car with my cartons full of notes and promised he would call if there were news from Ann.

It was a wonderful decision. Cummington, in the Berkshire foothills, offered peace and solitude as well as an opportunity that was rare for me—the chance to be with other writers. Besides being assigned a writing room in which I spent the day, I, like each of the residents, had chores to do. As I painted the wood stove, tilled the garden, and even shoveled cow dung, I felt the strength return to my body. My physical symptoms vanished, and feeling well brought emotional renewal. I was able to write again.

In my absence an early heat wave hit Connecticut. Paul left his office at two—when the tide was high—to wind surf. Arriving home to change, he found Annie in the kitchen. The blender was grinding to accommodate the load of ice cubes and piña colada mix.

"Guess who else is here?" she hugged Paul. "The celebrated Mr. Randy Slade!"

Randy raced in, dressed in striped pajamas and a necktie, threw his arms around Paul, and thanked him profusely for "the chance to spend a couple of fabulous days in the country."

Ann seemed defensive when Paul refused a piña colada and left to change his clothes. Randy tore around the house like a hyper-active child, banging chords on the piano, checking every chan-nel on TV, opening and closing the refrigerator, dashing from the living room out onto the deck.

Paul's business pressure was increasing, and he had been look-ing forward to a quiet evening. Returning downstairs, he found Randy stretched out on the sofa strumming Ellen's guitar.

"Ann," Paul said, "you can stay, of course. But I do not want Randy here. I have work to do at home. I need the house to be quiet."

Ann called Ellen to get my number in Cummington. "Mother," she said, "whose house is this, anyway? Didn't you and Paul pur-chase it together? Don't I have the right to bring a friend? You have no idea how hot it is in the city. We could hardly breathe in my apartment. Randy was so excited when I said he could come to my mother's house. I am stunned that Paul would be so ungracious."

"Have Paul call me, Annie. And you pick up on the kitchen phone. Let's have a three-way conversation."

When Paul returned from the beach, Ann did not suggest he call me. Instead she asked for a ride to the train. "I'm returning to the city with Randy."

Paul offered to wait for Randy to change his clothes. Randy and Ann looked puzzled. He had no other clothes. Randy wore his striped pajamas on the way to Westport and that is how he dressed on the train ride back to New York.

The following weekend my three weeks at Cummington ended. I said good-bye to newfound friends, I was delighted to have made great progress with the writing, and I hoped to return again.

Paul had dinner ready and fresh flowers on the kitchen counter. When I went to put my clothes away, I found the note Ann left propped against a perfume bottle on my bureau.

Mama—any chance of rescuing a daughter in distress? My apartment is in total shambles. I've forgotten how to work your method of starting to clean from one corner. More to the point, I can't even find the corner! Any help from a Mama would be mucho appreciated. I'll be home next Tuesday afternoon, for instance (unless that's too blatant a hint) and ready to follow your lead at precisely two o'clock.

Your loving but needy daughter—A.

As always she drew her initial A in the shape of a star.

Tuesday I loaded scrub brushes, sponges, Comet and Fantastic, a mop, the vacuum cleaner, and cleaning rags into Paul's little Opal. I made the trip down I 95 to Bruckner Boulevard, then onto the FDR Drive in little more than an hour, and parked in front of Ann's place at exactly two o'clock.

Weighted down with equipment, I felt breathless by the time I reached her floor. Gentle raps on the door of Ann's apartment got me no response. I pounded with the handle of the mop. Still not a sound. I left the cleaning supplies by her door and went back down the stairs to await her return.

Watching from the car, I began to notice a steady trickle of people heading into an abandoned building across the street. A young Hispanic boy beckoned at the doorway, and occasionally checked inside. More men than women, more blacks and Hispanics than whites, some teenagers, but mostly young adults entered the shelled-out structure and reappeared about ten minutes later.

A truckdriver coming down the road suddenly blasted his horn. I turned to see a man who looked like Ann's friend Randy standing in the middle of the street, offering the peace sign before he stepped aside. "Fuckin' hippie freak!" The driver raised his middle finger above the roof of the cab.

The pedestrian shrugged as if the driver were crazy. As he passed my car, I called his name and Randy ran to my car.

"Eleanor!" he kissed my hand. "Eleanor! Eleanor. What a surprise! How wonderful to see you!"

"Where is Annie, Randy? She didn't tell you that she asked me to come and help her today? I've been pounding on her door."

"Really? Well I betcha she just forgot. But don't you go worrying about that daughter of yours. Our friend Annie didn't go anywhere today. That crazy girl just sleeps so deep that I'd be locked out too if I didn't have me a key. So you just wait right here now till I go tell her that her mamma's come to visit."

I did not believe that Ann was inside. Twenty minutes later Randy returned to the street.

"I saw your cleaning supplies in the hall. Annie's place is a little too out of control at the moment for a mop and bucket to help. I don't even think a mamma could fix it. So anyway I'll get your stuff and put it in your car and then—" Randy stopped. He saw that the driver who had honked at him had parked a block away and was carrying stacks of boxes into a corner grocery. He left the motor running.

"Wait for me, Eleano-o-or," Randy called and sped away. I watched him leap up to the cab of the truck, and reach in through the window. Running back, he paused to toss something in the corner mailbox.

A little girl approached the driver. She pointed from his truck to the mailbox. The man took off his cap, and was stomping it in rage when Randy caught my arm.

"Don't worry. He'll get his keys back in a day or two," Randy said, pulling me into Annie's building and leading me up the stairs. I stopped on Ann's floor. Randy kept on climbing stairs until he turned and realized that I had not followed.

"Eleanor, I beg you. Come on up here a minute," he beckoned. "I was going to tell you to go home, but then I decided I should speak to you. But not near Annie's floor. God should have ears like your daughter."

What did this wild man have to tell me? I followed guardedly through a door at the top of the stairway and suddenly we stepped onto the rooftop of the building. The sun was intense. It took a moment of blinking before I realized that beyond the hundreds of rooftops and chimneys, spread a magnificent view of Manhattan.

The roof itself had no protective ledge, no railing. Just a long straight drop nine stories. Randy walked to the very edge. "Come over here. Don't stand there by the stairwell."

I had never been afraid of Randy. But now his head, his whole body, seemed to be pulsing to some inner stimulation. Why had he led me to the rooftop?

"I want to talk right here." I hugged the wall and considered running down the stairs.

"Gotcha—" Randy snapped his fingers. "Agoraphobic, right?" He came back and stood too close. His hand against the building blocked my path to the door. I felt trapped.

"Look, Eleanor, this is hard to say, but I think you ought to know"—he paused and looked around—"your daughter and I have gotten into certain drugs more heavily than either she or I intended. At first Annie kept us both in total control. We thought—you know—reality was for people who couldn't handle drugs." Randy smiled pleadingly. "Anyhow"—he cleared his throat—"the situation is now a bit ahead of us both."

I searched his eyes but they were unrevealing. It took a while to dare to ask. "What are you two using?" I held my breath.

"Heroin."

"Oh, no, God, no."

"Please don't be upset. That's just why she didn't tell you. She doesn't want to upset you. Annie is an alchemist. Really. She usually knows exactly what to take and when to stop. Just for a while we got ourselves carried away. So in another week or two we're going to New Jersey to a friend's place. We're gonna face the problem. Cold. No clinic. Nothing. Just two friends gettin' clean together.

"But for right now, Eleanor, you've got to understand. That girl of yours loves you too much to let you see what's been going on. She begged me to tell you to come back another time."

"I will not leave until I see her. I did not come to judge."

Randy shook his head and led the way downstairs. He turned his key in the lock.

"Is that you, Randy?" Ann called. "Did you get rid of my mother?"

"Shit, no." Randy looked at me.

"Oh, God," Ann said.

I was shocked and frightened by what had happened since the last time I saw Ann's place. The chairs and table from home, the beautiful African art, her stereo, even her dishes, pots, and pans—everything she had once so attractively arranged—was either missing or part of the pile of furniture, clothes, boxes, bags, and books heaped up to the ceiling. Underwear and sweaters dangled from open drawers. A bare mattress on the floor was strewn with Styrofoam cups, crumpled paper bags, and soda cans.

Ann stood with folded arms, leaning against the wall, watching my reaction.

"I don't want you to live this way another moment, Ann. I understand what's going on now. I want you to come home with me. I'll help you find a place to detox—Randy too, if he wants help."

"I did not want you in this, Ma." She shot an angry look at Randy. "We already have a plan to handle this ourselves. Tomorrow we are going to New Jersey. Just the two of us. That's the one and only way we intend to do it."

"Annie, no! Please, for God's sake, listen. You cannot do this by yourselves."

"Please leave now, Mother. I find your condescending attitude humiliating. You cannot make me go with you."

Later, answers to Ann's comment spiraled through my head, words I could not think of in her presence: Ann, do not tell me that it is I who humiliate you, when you humiliate yourself with needles. And if you truly do not want to hurt me, stop toying with your life.

I felt a failure for having been unable to persuade her to come home. I even fantasized returning with a hospital aide who would restrain my daughter and help me take her to a treatment center. Why was Randy, whom I had not trusted, more open with me than Ann? It was he who ended my confusion and denial. I was grateful to him for that.

* * *

As Dr. Robbins had suggested, I scheduled an appointment with Norman Itkowitz at Liberation Clinic, a store-front agency in a run-down part of Stamford. The windowsill hosted pots of dried-up philodendron. Cigarette butts spilled out of tinfoil ashtrays. The orange plastic chairs had burn holes. A small cork bulletin board displayed a list of A.M. methadone hours, an announcement of a new "dependents' group," and a faded newspaper article with the headline "Former Junkie Becomes Lawyer."

Norman Itkowitz strode into the waiting area. I liked the firmness of his handshake, the fast assessment in his light blue eyes. He looked both confident and boyish. My mother would have called him "apple-cheeked."

"What brings you here?" He led me to his comfortably cluttered office.

"First, I want you to see this picture of my daughter," I pulled Ann's high school graduation picture from my purse. "I cannot tell you more until I know you have a sense of Annie and the hopes we had for her future—the hopes she had for herself." Then the words tumbled out: brilliant student—budding anthropologist—something happened—Austen Riggs and Yale—and now the awful realization that she was using heroin.

"The fear of losing her is always with me now. I feel as if I have no right to my life until I find a way to save her. I need you to tell me how to help her."

"And I will tell you what I've had to say to many family members. Until she wants to stop herself there's nothing you can do." Norman passed me back Ann's picture. "Most people finally free themselves by giving up the effort to keep contact."

I shook my head. "That is not an option for me. At least not yet," I added.

Paul shook me gently when I cried in my sleep. One dream kept repeating: Ann was already dead but no one had the heart to tell me.

On Sunday I went to a meeting of Al-Anon, the group I had urged so many clients to attend. Over the years I had seen how

Al-Anon helped families like the Driscolls. Nothing in my training or in the therapy with Dr. Robbins offered what I needed now. I had to hear how other people dealt with loving an addicted person.

The meeting began with about sixty people reciting the Serenity Prayer:

> Grant me the serenity to accept the things I cannot change, the courage to change the things I can, and the wisdom to know the difference.

The first speaker told about her husband's emotionally abusive behavior after episodic drinking. "I used to think I had to take it, because I somehow caused it. This group has taught me the three Cs; I know now that I did not Cause it, I cannot Control it, and I cannot Cure it."

A man said, "I am learning how to separate the disease from the person. Now I can hate the disease. I do not need to hate my wife."

"I first came here to find out how to fix my daughter," a gray-haired woman said. "Now I'm here to help myself." People nodded knowingly.

Gradually I came to see that Al-Anon could serve as a special kind of toolchest for me, always available when needed. The Serenity Prayer became a mantra, to be repeated whenever I felt frightened or confused.

I turned to examine another part of my life. I had been on staff at the clinic for twelve years. It was time to move to another learning experience.

The Coalition for Children and Youth, an agency coordinating services for child protection, received a grant to interview and assess the needs of incarcerated mothers at the state prison for women. I applied for and got the job, which also involved contact with children whose mothers were imprisoned.

The work would be part time, allowing me three days a week to begin a private practice. I rented a small office in downtown

Westport, which afforded me a quiet place to write until my practice developed. But clients came more quickly than expected and writing had to be sandwiched in between my work as a therapist and the trips to the Niantic Correctional Center.

At first sight, the prison's redbrick buildings dotting the rolling farmland looked much like a college campus. Once inside, the duty officer chastised me. I had walked across a yellow line—which I had failed to notice—without waiting to be called. He then assigned me to a small room on the second floor. A pregnant eighteen-year-old was led in by a correction officer. Margarita's baby was due in a week. She had three more months to serve, and no one to take the newborn. I assured her that through Pat Blumenthal, director of the Coalition, the baby would have a nurturing interim home. Pickup would be arranged at the hospital four days after her delivery.

The second woman had yet to hear what had happened to her children the night she got arrested. Another begged for contact with her daughter, whose foster parents refused to accept her collect phone calls from the prison.

The last woman I saw had a teardrop tattooed just beneath her eye. Sharida had shot her battering husband. They had been on heroin together. She asked if I could trace the two young sons she had left with a neighbor who had apparently moved away. Sharida spoke of her early involvement with drugs.

Battered, streetwise women. Each asking for my help. I realized an agenda I had barely let myself acknowledge. I took the prison job to expand my work experience. But I was also hoping that working with addicted women would lead me to new ways to deal with Ann. I also feared that someday she might be arrested. I wanted to know what would happen. I felt certain she and Randy had not detoxed. She would have called if she had.

Late one June night, Randy did call. He told me he himself had successfully "kicked," but that Ann could not get "up" for her return to the Pyramid Club without returning to heroin. A month went by before Ann herself called. "Would you meet me at the two o'clock train tomorrow, Mom? I've already made arrangements to go to Silver Hill in New Canaan for rehab. They need to talk to you about the insurance."

I canceled my appointments with private patients. Nothing meant as much as getting Ann to a hospital. But she was not on the two o'clock train. Nor did she arrive at three. She finally got off the train that came in at four.

She was dressed in a long black sweater, too heavy for the muggy weather. Her thick black eye makeup heightened the gauntness of her cheeks. For the first time, Ann did not look clean. Her hair, her hands, even her face had a film of grime. She walked from the platform to the car as if her legs hurt, but insisted that she felt no pain.

I said I wished she'd called to let me know she'd changed the train time.

"I had no way to call," she said.

No matter now, I told myself. She will soon be in capable hands.

Ann dozed as I drove through the lush green countryside to Silver Hill. I was glad she would be in such a lovely setting. We arrived too late to see the intake worker together. Time only for a brief good-bye hug. I went to the financial office. Paul's help with insurance made the fifteen-hundred-dollar-a-week hospitalization something we could do for Ann.

I finished talking to the bookkeeper and headed out to the car, relieved to look back at the intake cottage and know she was safely inside.

But Ann was sitting in my car, puffing on a clove cigarette. A nurse had asked to search through her possessions. Ann refused to surrender her purse.

I could not take her home. She needed to be hospitalized. "Clean out your purse in the car," I said. "Use this paper bag. Just leave everything you don't want them to see. I promise not to look at the contents."

"I will not go back there to be humiliated." Ann crossed her arms and shook her head.

"Damn it, Ann, I feel set up by you—for all the wasted time and effort."

"Then drive me to the station," she said.

At the station, Ann jumped out and slammed the door before I fully stopped. Neither of us said good-bye. Not audibly. I said it in my heart. Maybe she did also.

> *I will not process myself*
> *through the Psycho-system again*
> *Expected to be acquiescent as a sheep*
> *hoping*
> *hoping for hope*
> *ready to accept whatever they would say*
> *about my problems*
> *buying the whole scam.*
> *I was so sincere.*
> *I believed.*
> *And so stupid.*
> *I believed.*
> *But I will not continue to believe*
> *anymore.*
>
> (DIARY ENTRY, OCTOBER 1984)

Paul asked me to go with him on a business trip to Sweden. We needed and deserved the time together. I informed my private patients and the prison that I would take a week off.

Ann called Ellen while Paul and I were away. Ellen drove her older sister back to Silver Hill. This time Ann allowed the nurse to check her purse. Ellen waited until Ann was shown to her room.

For the first two weeks, she was kept in isolation. She called and spoke about missing her old friend Tim, with whom she had gone to Africa. "Would you try to get his address from his mother and let him know I'm here? When I get out, I'd really like to see him again."

I found this request encouraging. Her relationship with Tim represented healthier times in her life. For Ann, too, I believed that seeking to reestablish contact with Tim augered hope for herself.

Tim's mother said that he was in France, working on a film-script. She would send him Ann's address at Silver Hill.

> Dear Tim,
>
> Greetings from your amigo, Typhoid Annie, writing to you from a beige-on-beige hospital room, currently transformed by the most dazzling luscious red roses I have ever seen, much less had the pleasure of receiving. All the nurses, experts in such matters, drop by to look and sniff. You couldn't have sent me a more welcome gift, nor more effectively extended your caring to a lonely friend.
>
> So here's the Ann scoop; less than sparkling health and vitality almost ever since post-Africa days. Thanks to ongoing insurance from both Mom and Paul, a chance for more long-term confinement than anything N.Y.C. had to offer. So here I am—rather more grateful now—having checked out the options to lay very, very low and serve my time.
>
> There's a good part that I hope you'll understand. I was into some pretty nasty drugs in the city. I've been using the time here to detoxify myself. Hooray! I've already started. So far, not too sick. I know it has to be a long haul, but when you return, if you should want to see me, I'll be one Clean Machine. Hallelujah.
>
> Tim dear, should you have the time, please keep in touch. It would mean so much to me now. All best wishes to you in every way, including filmwise.
>
> Thank you again for my lovely roses.
>
> Love, A.

Two weeks before her discharge Ann no longer needed methadone. Her doctor gave permission for a visit from Randy. I met him at the train station. We arrived at Silver Hill as staff and patients were leaving the activity buildings and walking up the winding driveway to the dining hall. Randy spotted Ann and leaped from my moving car. She ran directly into his arms.

"Randy-y-y-y-y!" she laughed.

"Annie-e-e-e-e," he screamed.

Every nurse, doctor, and patient within view of their reunion stopped to watch the wild young man lift the pretty girl and twirl her. Some of the same staff were heard to scream about an hour later, finding Ann and Randy in the shower, soaping each other like playful children.

At Ann's final discharge conference from Silver Hill, Paul and I expressed our fears that her return to the city would put her at risk of drug use again. We wanted her to stay in Westport at least for several months.

"I wish you wouldn't worry, Mom," Ann said. "I've been here for three months. I'm okay now."

Ann's doctor tried to assure us that she now understood how to take care of herself, and knew which persons and what substances had to be avoided. "Try not to worry about her return to New York," he said. "Ann has a career there. You have to let her go.

"Besides," he added, voicing almost exactly what her teachers used to tell me, "there is nothing this girl cannot do once she sets her mind to it."

Paul and I left her at the station. I gave her money to cover her rent and get her phone reconnected. She hugged us both and said how much she appreciated the chance we'd given her at Silver Hill.

During the next three months my therapy practice doubled. I spent two days each week at Niantic, and on the weekends worked on my new book. Ann seemed to have disappeared into the city. The time sped by without a word from her. There was no listing for the telephone she planned to get reconnected.

Christmas was coming. I had to track her down. The notes I mailed brought no response. I did not want to have the holiday without her.

> Street beat
> talking to my feet
> got me in rhythm again
>
> pulse of de city
> throb in my brain
> gotta get down to
> de street once again

Eleanor Craig

Back back
back in de city
back in de city again
My first abdication
since my relation
with dis here city began

Feeling peculiar
feeling sorta strange
walking de streets of
dis big town again

Street beat
comin through my feet
got me in rhythm again

(DIARY ENTRY, DECEMBER 1984)

Christmas
and Methadone

I readied the house for the holidays. The small room upstairs, hopefully, would be Ann's. I fixed the beds in the downstairs rooms for the three of Paul's five children who would be staying with us. We expected Doug Green and Trish, his bride, to take the shuttle from Washington where both practiced law. Alex—also a lawyer—was flying in from California, and Kathy would take time from graduate studies to drive down from Boston. Andrew, who worked with Paul, would drive over from Newtown Christmas day with his wife, Bettyann, and their two little sons, Scott and Adam. Peter, Paul's youngest, had joined the Peace Corps after college and was stationed in a village in Mauritania; he wrote to say that he would spend the holidays in Senegal.

When I attended workshops on blended families I felt very lucky that somehow we had beaten the odds. More often and openly than ever, experts were quoting research that suggested that couples with teenage children on both sides should either postpone marriage or forget it. But Paul's children, each with individual timing, were willing and able to become close to me, and I to them. Neither he nor I chose to force it. We had married without expectation of either instant gratification or commitment from our nine then unmarried children.

Together we mailed Channukah gifts to Pete, and Christmas presents to the Craig side of the family. Richard, Rosemary, and their darling baby, Zoya, were spending Christmas with Rosemary's parents in Red Wing, Minnesota. Billy and Nicola, who had married in St. Croix, were working in restaurants for the winter season and living close to Bill, my former husband. Paul had hired Ellen's husband, who spoke fluent Spanish, to represent his publications in Mexico. Ellen would spend Christmas in Mexico City with Charlie.

So although I was excited about the Green side of the clan coming home, a part of me felt keenly the absence of the Craig members. As I drove through evening traffic, I reviewed my plan to take the early-morning train to New York to hunt for Ann.

But when I walked into the kitchen at six-thirty there she was, standing at the counter, watching a creamy drink surging in the blender. The light glistening on her long thick hair, her stagey mascaraed eyes engulfing her pretty face, a blue-and-silver sweater opened over a silky lavender dress.

"Oh, Annie, what a great surprise! I can't believe it!" I scooped her into my arms.

It didn't matter any longer that she hadn't been in touch. Ann had come home for Christmas.

I poured myself a cup of instant coffee and sank into the old white wicker chair that serviced the round kitchen table. There was a moment's silence while Ann sipped on her frothy concoction, after which, almost shyly, our eyes connected and we both grinned simultaneously.

"When I was five," she said, "I used to look at the photographs of you, Mom, and try to smile exactly the way you smile."

"You still do," I said, but it was hard to focus on her generous lips. Ann's eyes still had a magnetic, almost hypnotic quality.

"Ma," Ann reached for my hand, "I know I let you down by not calling. Our hours are so different, and the longer I put it off, the harder it was to go to a pay phone. And I've been busy moving, too. I got a better place on East Ninth Street. I get the phone in next week.

"So I've been doing well, Ma. I hope that you and Paul will

come and see one of my shows soon. I am onstage alone now, every Sunday evening at the Pyramid. They call my night the Café Iguana and I write all the material for it.

"But most of all, I would love to have you and Ellie come on a Saturday and take part in the women's group I started. It's a new place, and it is really working to encourage women writers and artists. We call it Women in Limbo."

While I tried to keep up with her rapid speech, I found myself taking a kind of mental inventory of my oldest child's well-being. I wanted to believe that her light-colored dress was tangible proof that Annie now felt brighter, more hopeful than she had in all the years when, as though in mourning for herself, Ann had dressed only in black.

We talked for almost an hour, me telling Ann news about Richard, Billy, and Ellen and all the Green step-siblings, and about my work with families at the prison and with the children of incarcerated women, Ann talking about new friends she had made, about a showing of David's artwork, and about her own work in New York. She described a show she'd both written and performed in, parodying the "Family Feud" television show, with a Pyramid Club version of the Onassis clan—headed by Jackie—competing with the Snits, an "all-American family."

"It's being shown on cable TV, Ma. I hope you'll get to see it. I think you would be proud of me." Then there was a pause and Annie bowed her head.

"Ma, I—uh—I, I hate to have to tell you this, but I do not expect to stay through Christmas." She withdrew her hand from mine. I could not halt the stinging tears of disappointment that blurred my vision of her as she left the table and headed upstairs to her room. Instantly, I felt as though Ann were already miles away, as if she had somehow floated backward, far from any chance for me to reach her.

Over her shoulder, Ann promised she'd tell me more after making several phone calls. She was already curled up under the patchwork quilt in her old four-poster bed when I went up to call her for dinner.

"I'll eat later, Ma," she murmured. She did not leave her room until late the following morning.

Ann did not speak again about leaving before the holiday. When she asked me to go shopping with her the day before Christmas, I began to hope she would stay. All along Main Street, sales clerks in the crowded stores, strangers on the busy walkways paused to smile in response to the vivacious young woman in the dramatic wide-brimmed hat, paisley shawl, and long green flowing cape.

"Surprises, Ma," she said as she surged ahead of me into each store. "That's the fun of choosing presents. Finding some surprise—just exactly right for every person."

We didn't stop until the stores closed and our arms were loaded with bags of all sizes. By then it was snowing lightly and tiny golden Christmas lights outlined the branches of every tree on Main Street.

We stopped for a cup of seafood chowder at the Ship's Corner, stashing all the gifts under the cozy booth. I went to find the phone to see if Paul would join us. When I came back Ann was standing at the bar. She and the bartender were talking with such animation that I presumed he was a friend from high school.

"I thought some bloody Marys would warm us up, Ma," she said. No, she did not know the bartender.

The waitress put down Ann's drink first, a crystal mug of bloody Mary, out of which rose a pale green celery stalk. "The perfect drink for Christmas!" Ann grinned at her.

"Tommy," the waitress nodded toward the bar, "Tommy said he made yours double like you asked him. Even though serving doubles is against the law in Connecticut. He made you a double anyway."

When she left, Ann put her hand over mine. "I'm—uh—sorry, Ma. I guess I need a strong drink to be able to say this. I have to go back to the city early tomorrow morning. I cannot stay for Christmas dinner, or even to open the presents."

"But, Annie, why?"

"I—I'm—I'm sorry if it disappoints you. I didn't want to tell you, but a few weeks after Silver Hill I—I had to go back on methadone again, Ma. I was lucky to find a clinic that could take me. Some people go for months and months waiting to get on methadone.

"That's the reason that I never called, Ma. I didn't want not to tell you and I didn't want to disappoint you.

"I—uh—I'm so ashamed to need the methadone. I really had to beg to get the three-day supply they gave me so I could stay here at all. I—uh—I am so ashamed to—uh—to need it. But the clinic closes at noontime tomorrow. Having us come on Christmas Day is their way of checking up. And, Ma, I'm sorry but I— I cannot get through a day without it."

"Oh, Annie." I searched for a way to keep her home. "Why don't I drive you in? We could leave about ten—after everyone opens their presents. Then I'll wait so I can drive you back. I want you with us for Christmas, Annie. It would mean a lot to me."

"Oh, Ma," her eyes glistened, "would you really do that?"

The next morning Paul scrambled eggs while Ann and I made cranberry muffins and coffee. Paul put on our tape of the Vienna Boys' Choir singing "Adeste Fideles." Scott and Adam, our two little grandsons, seven young adults, and Paul and I shared a candlelit breakfast served buffet-style around the lighted Christmas tree.

Everyone loved Ann's funny, thoughtful presents. A special tree ornament for each person, engraved with names and "Christmas 1983." A subscription to *Windsurfer* magazine in recognition of Paul's new interest. Barrettes for my hair—barrettes with pullout pencils—"so what comes from your head goes directly to the paper," she'd written on the card.

Ann said she wanted to linger over her own gifts. She would open them all when we returned that afternoon.

At ten o'clock, she was still not ready to leave. I tried to press her to hurry, but she had locked herself in the bathroom and called through the door that she had to have more time to get ready.

Finally, at eleven, we left the house. Paul called time-out in the annual family football game being played in spite of our snow-covered field. He took me aside to speak. "Please don't speed. You know it's her own fault if you can't make it. It's almost impossible to get there in an hour."

Ann sat motionless and silent as we drove at as fast a speed as I dared. We pulled up in front of the clinic at just two minutes after twelve.

Ann leaped from the car before I fully stopped, dashed across Avenue A, and pulled at the metal door of a building so devastated looking that I assumed it had been condemned. Every window on all four levels had been boarded over. Ann continued to knock and tug on the door.

I watched from my car as a taxi ground to a jolting halt at four minutes after twelve. A black woman in a leather jacket and tight leopard-patterned pants jumped out and began pounding on the door with Ann.

"Open up, you motherfuckers!" the black woman screamed.

From opposite ends of the block, two white men ran until they too arrived at the doorway.

"Come on, come on," the bearded man in a jeans jacket pounded the door with both fists. The one in the ragged topcoat kicked so hard that he tumbled backward clutching his foot in pain. At that moment, the door opened outward.

An enormous black man, dressed in a long white tunic, stepped out onto the sidewalk brandishing a silver-colored baseball bat. "Ain't no use, you motherfuckers knockin'. You been tole that this here clinic close at twelve o'clock today. And the nurse that give out all that methadone this mornin', that little nursie probably already home right now, chewin' up her holiday turkey. Ain't her fault. Ain't my fault neither. Maybe some a you suckers gonna get some sense 'bout getting places when you s'posed to."

The black woman broke from the group, which had formed a circle around the man from the clinic. She yanked on the handle of the metal door with so much force, such a false expectation of success, that the effort caused her to fall backward onto the sidewalk.

"You wanna fuckin' die, girl?" the black man spun around and pinned her down on the cement, jamming his baseball bat into her now bared stomach like a rifle.

The man in the buttonless topcoat looked around as though the scene confused him. Then, wild-eyed, he dashed across the street, swerving to avoid the fender of my car. The first person he encountered, I felt for certain, would end up a victim in a mugging. Someone would be robbed so he could get himself street drugs. Helplessly, I watched in the rearview mirror until he disappeared around a corner.

Ann was still at the door, where she continued to plead with the attendant. The phrases I could hear sounded reasonable. "We only missed by a couple of minutes . . . Christmas day . . . a little leeway for people who tried pretty hard . . . other days we always come much later—four or five o'clock in the evening."

It hurt to watch the way the man's eyes narrowed, the smirk on his face as he surveyed my daughter from her head down her narrow body to the tips of her boots and up again. I wanted to rush out to help her, to say to the man, "For God's sake stop playing games and give these people the methadone!" But I knew Ann would turn on me if I intervened.

Suddenly, he dropped the bat and raised his hands in the air as if he were under arrest. "Little junky woman wanna hold me up? Make me feel real bad with all that white girl bullshit? You think twelve o'clock ain't twelve o'clock just on account you a honkey?"

I held my breath as the man picked up the bat again, and spun around pointing it at Ann, the black woman, and then the bearded man. "You suckers shoulda asked ole Santa give you some kinda timepiece, 'cause one thing you gonna learn is gettin' on the clock. Off the horse and on the clock. You hear me? 'Gwan now—have yourselves a few little cramps. Make you remember good when ole Santa come back next year."

He strutted down the street while Ann helped the black woman to her feet. The little group stared after him, the black woman screaming, "Motherfucker, motherfucker," and then they all dispersed.

Ann leaned in the window on my side of the car. "I'm sorry, Ma. I realize that it's my fault. You rushed so hard to get here."

"Annie, whom can we report that guy to? The police? Some kind of public health commission? Is there a—"

"Stop, Ma." She put her head on my arm. "The city doesn't care about us. I'm sorry, Ma—after all your efforts—now I can't come home after all."

"Annie, please get in; let's see if there's another solution." I felt desperate not to lose her so soon.

Aimlessly, we drove around the devastated blocks, past heap after heap of rubble where buildings once had stood. Finally I said, "Why not come home with me, darling? Maybe we could get you some Valium, or some sedative to hold you till tomorrow. I don't want to leave you here on Christmas day."

"You don't understand, Ma. Valium or a sedative wouldn't help me. There is only one way I could come home, Ma, and that is if I could buy some street drugs. I swear to you that I will be back on methadone tomorrow. I just have to get through today."

My gut reaction was to say good-bye; drugs were not an option I could accept. But as I turned to look at her, my own need to try to help her and not lose her on this Christmas Day, took over. I could not bear the thought of driving off alone, knowing it could be weeks, even months before I would hear from her again.

"Where do we go?" I asked.

Ann directed me to a corner on Avenue C. There she got out of the car, walked down the street, and turned right. The moment she disappeared from my line of vision I felt crazed for being in such an unholy position.

I saw a black boy, only about eleven, pop out from the doorway of the shell of a building, whistle twice, then disappear again. Down the street, a boy about the same age suddenly appeared from around a corner where Ann had gone. The second boy whistled. I watched the first boy dash down the block and as abruptly as they had appeared, the two youths vanished together.

I tried to ward off violent images. What if they were attacking Ann? Could I ask God to protect her, when I knew she was off buying drugs?

Twice a patrol car cruised by. The first time the policeman turned to look at me. The second time I saw him note the license plate on the car. Could Ann have been arrested?

In an hour, only two people walked down the forsaken avenue. Where had she gone? Why did it take so long? Could the drug cause her to forget that I was waiting? What if she overdosed? How would I find out? I heard a siren in the distance. I was afraid to go looking for her. If she came back and I were gone, she would disappear again.

Somehow Ann returned from a different direction, approaching from behind the car. I was startled when she jiggled on the door I had so carefully locked.

"Mom, I can't thank you enough. That was awful. I thought I would never have to do it again. I know it was awful for you, too."

As I drove out of the Lower East Side, back onto the FDR Drive paralleling the welcome brightness of the river, Ann described her experience, telling it as though she were unaware of my presence, but needing to review it for herself.

". . . Past the spotters . . . just little boys those dealers use to protect themselves . . . little boys pointing the way for the junkies . . . little kids getting paid off with heroin . . . the teenaged kids who guard the bombed-out building where the stuff was . . . never know which building . . . climbing through a hole they made . . . spotters giving flashlight signals . . . only the dealer protected . . . then I had to crawl across the plank . . . black space . . . the bucket comes down on a rope . . . down from a hole in the ceiling . . . put my money in the bucket . . . the big man pulls the rope up . . . when the money is right, he sends the bucket down again . . . the drugs, the works, in the bucket . . . the heroin."

As she told about getting the drugs, Ann crawled over the front seat to lie down in back. She continued with her halting story. I was horrified by the risk and degradation and by the thought of how often she must have done this. Ann's words slowed. Finally she stopped talking. I could see in the rearview mirror that she was sleeping. Somehow seeing her curled up in the backseat of the car, as if she were a little girl again, was helpful. I knew where my child was. I would bring her home with me. She would have food and her own clean bed to sleep in tonight.

At home Ann said she was too exhausted to come down for dinner. As she headed for her bedroom she could only mount the carpeted stairs by holding on to the railing and pulling herself one step at a time.

"I guess the methadone really wipes her out," Paul glanced at me in concern, then began to carve the holiday turkey. As they helped me in the kitchen, each of my daughters-in-law and each of Paul's children extended comforting hugs to me without refer-ring directly to Ann. I was not ready to admit to Paul or anyone in the family the terrible choice I had made in order to bring her home again.

That night I kept getting out of bed to check on her. Ann lay draped across her bed, arms and head dangling over the side. I stood at the doorway watching, waiting to make sure that she was really breathing. Each time I went back to my own room wondering whether she would be there in the morning.

Ann's old high school friend David Barton called at seven-thirty, while Paul and I were having coffee. An artist, David lived in a loft in the city but had spent the holiday in Westport visiting his parents. He could drive Ann back to New York.

David picked her up at nine o'clock. Ann had had no time for breakfast. She left wearing the clothes she had slept in. Either she or David would pick up her Christmas presents later, she promised. She hugged me and thanked me again, "For yesterday, for everything, Ma."

Ann waved from the car. Watching them drive off, I felt both fear and sadness. For the third time that I knew of, Ann was on a methadone maintenance plan. Neither hospitalization nor the previous outpatient clinic had freed her from addiction. I felt a rush of guilt for having driven her to Avenue C.

When Paul left, I went into the living room to gather up Ann's presents. I knelt by the box with the fur-lined boots she had raved about the day we shopped together. A sob caught in my throat. I had been so eager to see her open my present. I finally pulled

myself up and left her gifts as she had, wrapped and spread out
underneath the Christmas tree.

Do you fear that you've lost control again
Riding through a twilight of greed.
Do you find yourself lurking in shadows
Looking for what you need?

Are you riding the dark horse, baby—
Old Satan taking you for a ride?
Don'tcha wonder if you'll ever slow down again—
Ain'tcha scared of that final slide?

(DIARY ENTRY, DECEMBER 1984)

T H I R T E E N

Spiraling

On New Year's Eve, the other children phoned but Ann did not.
She sent an envelope full of announcements and reviews:

> Ma, just to let you know what I'm up to. Miss you.
> Lots of love to all. A.
> P.S. Doing well on the meth.

> Come Celebrate a Replay of the Family Feud—
> Starring Ann Craig
> and
> Featuring the Snit Family from Centralia, Missouri
> vs. the Family Onassis

> The groundbreaking celebration of the
> Lower East Side Polygon
> presented by MC: Ann Craig

> ". . . dressed in huge veiled hats, flowing scarves,
> and larger than life costumes, and with outlandish
> eyeliner, Craig arrived in New York from Con-
> necticut four years ago and soon became in-
> strumental in the East Village performance art
> scene . . ."

I read the ads and article to Paul. "She's really on her way," he said.

Late in March, 1985, New York City Mayor Ed Koch ordered a major sweep of the Lower East Side. Hundreds of addicts were to be rounded up and jailed. I wanted to believe Ann's note, that she was doing well on methadone. But my work at the women's prison reinforced the fear that Ann could be arrested.

"I always hated needles," a young addict told me. "But once I did it, I was always chasing the next one. The feeling was so incredible. Like you can't scream any louder," she said. "I'll be shooting up the day I get released. Once a person gets the ultimate, ain't nothing gonna substitute."

Ann's phone, which I gave her money for, was never reconnected. I went to the city hoping I would see her. The hole in the door of her apartment filled me with foreboding. The lock had been punched out. Two men patching cracks in the ceiling had never seen the former tenant. Her furniture and clothes were gone.

I went by Mercy House, hoping, dreading, to see her among the homeless. Instead, I spotted Sophie sitting on the stairs. "Remember me, Sophie? Your friend Annie's mother? You gave me a pretty scarf. Have you seen Annie, Sophie?" I handed her five dollars. Sophie grabbed the money. Then she peered at me suspiciously and began to make a hissing sound.

The Pyramid Club was bolted up. I walked two blocks past a woman curled up in a doorway but I knew I had to turn around. She was wrapped in a black coat and wearing a beret like Ann's. I went back to look closer. Her skin was dark and wrinkled. She opened her eyes and put out her hand. I gave her money. Then she mumbled, "Can you take me home?" Ann would not have said that.

In April, when Paul and I came home from a Seder dinner with our friends the Sarkins, Ellen met us at the door.

"Where were you, Mom? I've been here an hour. Randy has

been calling my house constantly. He says Ann is in terrible trouble. She's in some kind of drug-related coma."

Just then, our phone rang. It was Randy, who said Ann would not stop jabbing needles into her arm. "I begged her to stop. And now she's slumped on the floor, completely unresponsive."

"For God's sake, Randy," I screamed, "call an ambulance and get her to a hospital. Call me from the emergency room. I will come as soon as you tell me where."

Paul and Ellen and I waited together. I huddled on the couch, feeling chilled and shaky, sending silent prayers to my daughter. Ellen sat beside me. An hour passed with no word from Randy.

"Ann has to be alive," Ellen said. "We would have heard if she weren't." We held hands as Paul called city hospitals. No emergency room had treated a patient named Ann Craig.

Paul slumped over the kitchen table, holding his head. "Where in God's name would he have taken her?"

Ellen began to weep. I held her and we cried together.

Paul put his arms around us both. "I agree with Ellie," he said. "Someone would have called by now if Annie didn't make it."

The phone rang.

"What happened?" I cried.

"Honest, Eleanor, I couldn't get back to you any sooner. Annie wouldn't let me. She came out of the coma right after I talked to you. She begged for more cocaine and mescaline. She said I had no right to stop her, that she was ready to die. I had to get her walking. I took her out for food and coffee. I pleaded with her to call you. I told her you would be so anxious. Oh, Eleanor, you know how furious she gets. 'My mother is *not* to be involved,' she said."

"My God, Randy, what kind of craziness is that? Ann was ready to die and I was not to be involved?"

"She's asleep here on the floor beside me. But you don't have to worry. She is breathing normally now."

I hung up the phone feeling so helpless and angry it was difficult to repeat the conversation.

Paul said the time had finally come to draw the line. "Her behavior will kill you if you don't."

Last night on the twilight steed
Riding wild through a nightmare of greed
Wild horses stampede in my brain
Crazy ride to outdistance the pain

(DIARY ENTRY, APRIL 1985)

Paul shook me gently. "You were grinding your teeth again. What is it?"

I had dreamt of trying to take Ann somewhere, but I could not find the key to start the car. I finally pulled it from a kangaroolike pouch on my abdomen. But the key would get us nowhere. All the teeth were broken.

"Paul, what if I die first? Who will look for her then?"

"I will," he said. "I promise."

Two days later I heard directly from Ann. "I have to ask a favor, Ma. If you would loan me sixty dollars I could get into an inner-city drug rehabilitation center."

"I am not the Red Cross," I said. "How can you call and ask me to help after what you put us through?"

"Ma, please. I lost all my perspective. I had a problem, and it left me mighty vulnerable to the old addictions. I felt such a twisted sense of reality. No way out. Nothing but despair."

"I do not understand that, Ann." I had no tolerance for her vagaries. "What exactly was the problem?"

Sometime in January 1985, she had begun to experience the soaring fevers she'd had on returning from Africa. Fevers of unknown origin. Too ill to stay alone, she went to live with her friend David, who shared his loft with two talented filmmakers, Susan and Melissa.

Ann acknowledged threatening to disappear if David were to let the family know she was ill. She promised to call home as soon as she felt better. In spite of her fevers she had to perform at the Pyramid on weekends, or she would be replaced. Nonetheless, if I had known she was ill, I would have tried to prevent her from performing.

One evening, on her way to work, she began seeing people on the street wearing her unmistakably identifiable clothing—her jeweled velvet robes, the tiered lace skirt she used as a mantilla. Panic-stricken, she raced back to her old neighborhood. In the months she'd been at David's, she'd never thought to pay her rent. Her door was broken, the rooms completely bare. A woman saw her weeping and confirmed that the landlord had tossed her books, clothing, and furniture onto the street. Strangers had been picking through Ann's possessions for days. There was nothing left to salvage. Frantically she searched through refuse containers, in junk stores, at bookstalls. Only one thing mattered. She had to find her African diaries. Someone might have saved them, if only for the leather bindings.

"When I realized that my diaries were gone, Ma, I got even sicker. All my hopes for myself seemed lost. Those diaries were my past and future—all the notes for the book I planned to write someday."

She went to Randy's rented room with what she thought was a lethal supply of drugs and an unfinished letter.

> Mamma,
>
> I am desperately sad, devastated about everything I have irrevocably lost—all my possessions thrown onto the street by my landlord. People have walked by me wearing my clothes and costumes. Most devastating of all, my African diaries are missing. For weeks I have been searching, praying I would find them. I feel defined by my loss. (Please note, by my fault, mine, no question.) What do I have to say to you, all of you: I have nothing to share but my overwhelming grief and embarrassment.
>
> For so long the experts you trust have tried to brace you for my eventual absence. Your awareness of the pain I feel would force you to take steps to "save" me. Better we stay apart and

I sent the sixty dollars for Ann to be admitted to the rehabilitation center. At worst it would buy more drugs. At best, she might be safely hospitalized while the citywide crackdown continued.

When I called the city clinic to ask if she were admitted a woman responded that such patient information was confidential. On my third call she finally said, "That girl be jivin' you, honey.

Ain't nobody come in here fast as that. If she get in before a month, she be one of the luckies. Far as the city concerned, your girl be just another addict, and saving a addict's life ain't got no kinda priority. So keep on prayin' for her, honey. Ain't nothin' more us mammas can do. My boy Rodney, he died a overdose. Two years since then, they the only peace that boy ever give me."

Ann called that afternoon. "Mom, I am about to walk through the door into the lockup rehabilitation unit. I'm scared, Ma, and I wanted you to wish me luck before I do it."

No matter what her reason, even simply to avoid arrest, Ann was about to get help. I could not resist feeling hopeful. "I do wish you luck. Hold your head up high and walk right in there, Annie. My heart is with you always."

We could not visit, or even make contact by phone. But Ann did send a letter:

> Mom, I know you're working awfully hard. Ellie wrote me about the heavy schedule you have taken on—but do try to get in some time for yourself. Have you had any chance to walk on the beach like we used to?
>
> If you'd like, I would care very much to hear about what's up with you—your work, your writing, your loving and living.
>
> Whatever, I always aim my greatest love to you.
>
> A.

Ann came home in August to celebrate her "graduation" from the program. She was thin but bright and energetic. Paul gave her editorial work at his office, and she seemed in no hurry to return to the city. We began to talk about her taking courses to get the few last credits she needed to complete her degree.

At summer's end, Ann asked if she and Randy might borrow my car for a weekend camping trip to a state park in Rhode Island. I said yes, explaining to Paul how much I wanted to treat her as I would our other children.

Ann expressed the same excitement I remembered from her first Girl Scout camp-out. She and Randy packed sleeping bags, a rented tent, and cooking equipment into the car. At seven on a balmy night she called to say that they had put up the tent, cooked bluefish over an open fire and even roasted marshmallows.

"Thank you both so much, Ma. It's so healthy to be here."

Randy took the phone. "This girl and I feel just like little kids. It's kinda like the frosting on Annie's great recovery."

"I guess I was wrong not to trust them," Paul shook his head.

The Rhode Island State Police called at midnight. Ann had crashed into a tree on the state camping grounds. She said she swerved to avoid a chipmunk. The Emergency Medical Service ambulance had taken her to the hospital. She was conscious. The automobile was totaled.

Her brothers Richard and Billy drove with me to Rhode Island General Hospital. A surgeon explained that he had wired her broken jaw. He did not prepare us to see that she had lost her front upper teeth. Nor that her eyes were flat and distant again.

We picked up Randy at the campsite. Their tent was strewn with stubs of marijuana joints. A blackened spoon, a straight razor, a small mirror, and rolled-up dollar bills were spread on one of the sleeping bags. I expressed my shock and disappointment at having thought I could trust them. Randy cheerily acknowledged having "partied too much." Ann, still groggy from the surgery, seemed to have no recall of the night's events.

Richard drove. I sat beside him. Billy and Randy shared the backseat. Richard, Billy, and I were too angry to respond to Randy's efforts to converse. Ann curled up in the back of Paul's car. Billy covered her with the sleeping bags. When she moaned, he reached back to stroke his sister's head.

Ann endured painful and extensive dental work. But her mouth was never the same. Just as teeth do not come back, I finally stopped believing that the "old Annie" I so yearned for—the girl so full of dreams and promise—would ever return.

Her dental work was still in progress when Ann returned to New York to do a benefit show at the Pyramid Club for her good friend and fellow performer, Tron, who was hospitalized with AIDS. David called to say that Ann's performance was one of her most brilliant. The show raised thousands of dollars. But Tron died the following day.

Ann stayed in the city. She missed two dental appointments. One month later, David took her to a hospital. Ann had hepatitis. She tested negatively for AIDS. After a four-week hospitalization, she returned to our house to rest.

Paul bought her the sewing machine she asked for. I took her for rides into the countryside and tried to keep her well supplied with books. But we told her we could not continue to be available to nurse her back to health, if she persisted in living so self-destructively. It was too painful for us.

Then the fevers returned, hitting 105 degrees. She resisted the idea of rehospitalization, but agreed to go if I would let her spend just one more night in her own bedroom. The doctor said he would admit her through the emergency room at nine the following morning.

Sometime during the night Ann called David, who picked her up while we were sleeping. When I woke up to get her breakfast I found her note on the kitchen table: "Mother, can't you see that coercion causes hostility? I do not want another hospitalization. Love, A."

She was sick and she was gone again.

> *I can leave anytime that I want to*
> *I can walk out that door anytime*
> *that I feel I got to*
> *I can leave you*
>
> *Tap a tap hear the sound of my footsteps*
> *Tap a tap hear me crossing the floor*
> *Tap a tap, that's the sound of my heartbeat*
> *All I hear is my hand on the door.*

(DIARY ENTRY, JANUARY 1986)

Finding Ann

Richard called from Washington on April 21. His boss had given final confirmation that he and his family would be transferred to Hong Kong. I expressed my joy at his promotion, but I knew I would miss them, miss my monthly visits to him and Rosemary, to dearest Zoya, who had just turned five, and little David, almost three. Yet even stronger than the sense of loss was my compulsive need to contact Ann. The prospect of Richard's departure filled me with fear that if Ann did not come home in May when he and his family came to say good-bye, he might never see his sister again.

I had to find her, regardless of how David tried to put me off. Every time I called, he was friendly but evasive.

"Ann? Uh—no, Ann isn't here right now. In fact, you just missed her."

"I think she said she was going out of town this week."

"Just saw her yesterday. I don't know when I'll see her again."

Was she sitting right beside him as he lied to me, nodding her appreciation for his cooperation? It had happened so many times before—to me, to her father, to her brothers and sister—David saying Ann was out or sleeping and that he would surely tell her to call. But she never did. Right up until the night of Richard's farewell party, I had failed to reach her.

Bill and Nicola drove down from their new home in New Hampshire. Ellie, whose husband was away, arrived with baby Charlie. Paul prepared steamed clams. I stuffed lobsters with crabmeat, Richard's favorite dinner.

When we toasted to Richard's and Rosemary's great adventure, Ellen announced that "When you come back there'll be a new addition in the family."

"Make that two," Billy grinned, his arm circling Nicola.

I looked at the radiant young faces around our candlelit table. David and Charlie crawled into my lap. I felt very blessed. My fear for Ann's well-being never completely left me, but I had forced myself to learn not to let it overshadow precious moments with my other children.

Cleaning up the kitchen after dinner turned into a replay of times past—family renditions of Beatle songs, show tunes, including fancy footwork to "Steam Heat" and "Hernando's Hideaway," and by popular request, the medley of World War Two songs that Paul and I began with "Any Bonds Today."

After Zoya, David, and Charlie were tucked into beds, I reviewed my fruitless efforts to contact Ann, without conveying my mounting sense of urgency—the fear that time could be running out. It was Ellen who said, "I keep dreaming about her, Mom. I dream that she is falling."

At 10:00 P.M. Richard decided to make one last call to David.

"Hong Kong! Ann will be excited for you," David said. "Unfortunately, I don't have any way to reach her. She is doing some house-sitting for a friend—I don't even know the person's name, but as far as I'm concerned, it's pretty good timing. She told me it was a ground-floor apartment. Ann has not been feeling well. She was having trouble getting up the many flights of stairs here. You know how steep loft stairs are . . ."

Hearing Richard reconstruct his conversation with David, I became convinced that David had been lying—not about her health, but about her staying at anyone else's apartment. I knew too well from countless efforts to find her that Ann no longer had contact with anyone but David. People who had once pursued her as an entertainer had long ago stopped calling, assuming she had chosen to drop out from the club and cabaret scene. Occasionally, a few old friends called my home on the chance she might have come back to Connecticut, or that I would know her whereabouts.

David said she was not feeling well. I felt certain that if I were going to find my daughter I would find her in a hospital. Paul, who had lived in the city, dictated names of places to try.

My first call was to Mount Sinai. "I believe my daughter may have been admitted," I said. "Her name is Ann Craig."

"I do not find her name. She may have already been discharged. What was her date of admittance?"

The male receptionist at Saint Claire's admitting office said, "Our computer is down. If you want to hold on I'll sort through the names by hand. . . . Sorry to have kept you waiting so long. We have no one by that name on record."

By the time I got through to Beth Israel Hospital, Ellen had carried sleepy little Charlie out to her Jeep. Only Richard and Bill remained in the kitchen.

"Patient's phones don't ring after ten P.M.," a woman answered.

"What is the room number?" I asked. "I'd like to call her in the morning."

"Craig, Ann, let's see . . ."

I could feel my pulse throbbing in my eardrums.

"Ask for room ten-sixteen. The operator will connect you after seven-thirty in the morning."

"How do we know it's our Ann?" Billy said. "There could be lots of Ann Craigs in the city."

Paul and I drove Richard, Rosemary, and the children to the airport limousine at 6:00 A.M. "It's hard to go not knowing what is happening to Annie," Richard said as we hugged good-bye. Perpetuating a superstition of my mother's, something she called her Irish Good-bye, I waved until Richard and his family could no longer see me, but I shut my eyes instead of watching their limousine turn the final corner to the thruway.

Paul and I had breakfast at a restaurant called the Family Diner.

He left me at the railroad station. "Do you feel certain the patient will be Annie?" he asked.

"Very certain."

"Then give her my love."

There was an armed guard just inside the hospital door that faced out to Sixteenth Street. Beyond him, in the lobby, four women waited in attendance behind a circular reception desk. I was certain Ann would have requested no visitor other than David, so I could not risk announcing my arrival. Had I come this close only to be stopped now?

I spotted the ladies room on the left side of the lobby, and I hurried as though it were my only destination. When each of the receptionists seemed occupied, I scurried from the ladies room across the lobby to the bank of elevators, hoping the guard would assume I had already gotten the visitor's pass.

The tenth-floor nurses' station was the hub from which four corridors radiated. I had no idea which route might lead me to room 1016. The first hall I chose turned out to have only rooms numbered in the twenties. The nurses at the station still had their heads bent over records, but I worried about attracting their attention if I had to pass them again.

The second hallway I chose led to room 1016. A yellow paper lettered in black marker was taped to the closed door. All visitors for Ann Craig must report to the nurses' station.

I took time for a silent prayer, then tentatively opened the heavy door and stepped into a four-bed ward. The balding woman on my left seemed comatose, eyes shut and her toothless mouth ajar. Lines of blood and fluid dripped from an overhead stanchion into her withered arm. The looseness of her hospital gown revealed a bony chest. Beyond her writhed a naked white-haired woman, coos and grunts accompanying her gestures of masturbation. To my right a woman with one drooping eye scribbled sentences on her Formica bed tray with neither pen nor pencil. Her index finger was her writing tool. The fourth bed was screened off from my vision. Anxiously, I tiptoed around the barrier to find out whether my daughter was the occupant.

When our eyes met, a fat, grimy woman shook her fist at me.

"Margarita, get outta here, Margarita," she raged. "Why you no let my Tony come to see his momma? Why my. . . ."

Oh, God. I wanted to run back to the street and let the rain wash over me. Then, I turned back to the first bed and looked again—looked at the old woman getting blood. Could that comatose woman getting the transfusion be my Annie . . . ? Could my own child be beyond my recognition?

I stood at the foot of her bed. Her name was taped to the footboard. "Annie, Annie, I'm here," I whispered, moving closer to her head. "I just want to be with you, dear. It's Mother, Annie, and I love you."

Suddenly her eyes opened wide. "Didn't you see the sign?" she pointed, her bony finger shaking. "I told the nurses someone in my family might pull this, and if you do not leave this minute everyone here is prepared to call the police. *Get out! Get out of here this minute!*"

Holding back a rush of tears, I left the room. A young blond nurse was in the hallway. I said, "May I speak to you? I'm Ann Craig's mother. I have to talk to someone about her."

She led me to two battered wooden chairs across from the bank of elevators. I did not want to sit down.

"Help me, please! I need to know about Ann. Her family loves her very much. We have been looking for her for a long time now. I just saw her and I can't believe she can get well again. She looks as though she is dying. You have got to tell me. Is that true? Is my daughter dying?"

"Ann is an adult, Mrs. Craig. She is thirty-four years old, and she has a right to patient confidentiality."

"But you would be making a terrible mistake!" I pleaded. "Ann would not want to be separated from her family now—not when she needs us—not unless she thinks that we could not accept her illness, that she has something so terrible that she cannot let us help her."

"I am sure I would feel the same way you do, if I had a daughter who was ill, Mrs. Craig, but she is getting good care here."

"Her family has a right to be with her, a right to know about her illness." I could not bring myself to say the word I was and had been thinking. AIDS. AIDS. AIDS. Had I finally found her when there could be no hope?

"Ann is getting IVs now," the nurse spoke quietly. "Then we will be releasing her to outpatient care. Our follow-up is very good at Beth Israel."

"Will they find her a place to live? You know they can't do that! And she cannot even get up the stairs where she is living. Please. I am a psychotherapist. I must talk to someone about the mental health part of this. Ann must be suffering aberrations not to let her family help her now. Is there a social worker I can speak to?"

"The social worker is not in on Wednesday."

"There must be a psychiatrist—someone I can talk to."

"I'm afraid none of the mental health staff would be available to speak with you today, Mrs. Craig. Tomorrow you might try to reach the social worker by telephone. I'm sorry, you will have to leave now. I have to get back to my patients."

Just then there was a clatter. The nurse and I both turned in the direction of the sound. A skeletal patient, in hospital gown, with gauze pads on her head, was weaving her way down the hall, her trembling hand causing the wheeling stanchion to which her tubes were connected to rattle as she pushed it along.

"Mother," Annie's feverish eyes seemed to take up half of her shrunken face. "Mother, if—if—if I sp—speak to you here, will—will you promise to go away?"

"Yes, I will do whatever you ask me if you will just let me talk with you."

The nurse walked away, calling back, "I'll be right at the station if you need me, Ann."

"I didn't want you to see me this way, Mother," Ann's voice trembled and her body shook violently.

She reached for me and fell into my arms, and still the words she spoke were fiesty. "I am an embarrassment to you. You have told me that my whole life has been a waste."

"Oh, Annie, Annie. I have never said that your life was a waste. That's not how I feel at all." I kissed her fevered cheek. "You have helped so many people. You mean so much to me and everyone in our family. How could your life be a waste? Here, let me help you back to bed, dear. Please, Annie, let me sit beside you for a while."

Slowly, with my arm supporting her, Ann and I returned to room 1016. She sank into the pillow and closed her eyes. I watched in silence as two nurses came in to reconnect another plastic unit of blood.

Thank God, I thought, watching them change the needle in her arm, thank God they do not have on rubber gloves. No, whatever she had, it could not be AIDS. Not with nurses changing needles without protecting their hands. And if she did not have AIDS, perhaps she could get well.

"May I speak to you?" I followed her nurses into the hallway.

"I'm sorry," the gray-haired nurse answered. "Ann was very specific in requesting the staff not to speak to anyone regarding her condition. We all are obliged to respect those wishes."

Helplessly, I stayed by her bed for an hour, watching the stream of blood in one tube, the beads of milky fluid in another course through their channels into my daughter's arm. The silence was broken by heavier footsteps than the nurses. I turned to watch David pale as he entered and saw me by Ann's bedside.

"Don't worry, David, Annie knows I am here."

Her eyes remained shut. "My—mamma—" Between each word she halted a moment. "My mamma wouldn't stop until she found me. It is all right, David, she can stay here."

"David." When I stood to greet him, the handsome young man towered over me. "I think I understand it, David. I think I understand now why you could not tell me."

"She just did not want you to see her until she was looking better." David sounded anguished. "But I kept telling her after every time you would call, I kept telling her, 'Ann, your mother must really hate me.' "

"Mamma," Ann spoke without opening her eyes, "those times when I made David lie to you, sometimes he would get off the phone and cry. He didn't want to do it, did you, David?"

"I'm just glad that your mother is here now." David sat on the edge of her bed, cupping her wasted fingers in his generous hand.

"I didn't know how to feel about you, David," I said. "I was always grateful that you—that someone—seemed to know where Ann was. But I have to tell you there were times when I'd get so frustrated hearing your excuses that I did blame you for standing in the way of me finding my daughter. I even wondered whether I could get a court to order you to let me see her."

David turned from Ann to me, his eyes brimming with tears. "I'm sorry."

"I'm sorry, too." I reached across Ann's bed to clasp his hand. "I understand now."

Ann blinked at us in puzzled silence. "Mom," she finally said, "if David didn't tell you, how did you know where to find me?"

I told them about calling all the hospitals, a story Ann later told and retold to everyone who would listen. "My mamma called every hospital in New York City until she found me. . . ."

Ann and I both watched as David unpacked two bags full of presents: A plastic container with a bit of salmon he himself had sautéed in butter. A soft blue nightgown chosen for Ann by his mother. A flowered bottle of Yardley lotion with which he tenderly massaged her needle-bruised arms. Handsome David, all dressed up in jacket and tie, treating Ann as though she were still as beautiful as she had been.

Before I left, I asked Ann to come home and let me take care of her until she was feeling stronger.

"I have to go back to the apartment first, Ma. But I expect to be out tomorrow. I will call you, I promise."

I wanted to believe her, wanted to believe that no matter what the future held, we had finally reconnected. But on the elevator I was racked with the grief of finding her in such terrible condition. Suddenly I felt an arm across my shoulder.

"My father is in intensive care," a gray-haired woman in a belted raincoat said, holding me tightly. "Who is it for you, hon?" She led me off the elevator to a nook by the pay telephone. "Don't hold it back. Just let it go."

I sobbed on the woman's shoulder. For that moment she loved me and I loved her.

Then the stranger picked up her paper shopping bag.

"I'm gonna pray for your daughter," she said.

"And I will pray for your father."

We made our separate ways through the revolving door.

Ann did leave the hospital the next day. I kept in touch with David, who said she slept as much as eighteen hours a day. "I'm driving to Cape Cod to house-sit for some friends," he said. "As soon as Ann is feeling better we are hoping she can fly up to Hyannisport to join me."

It seemed preposterous to me that Ann would be able to get to the airport and take a plane to David. But she did. He called to say they went out for a lobster dinner. She still felt weak but was resting a lot.

I felt a little crazy telling Paul about David's phone call. There seemed almost no reality between the daughter I saw in the hospital and the person David described.

Ten days later Ann was back in New York and spoke to me directly.

"Could you come into the city tomorrow, Mom? There's something I want to talk about."

My appointments no longer had priority. This was, I hoped, my chance to bring my daughter home with me. We set the time for my arrival. Noon.

At 11:00 P.M., an hour after the first call, Ann phoned again. "I've thought it over." Each word came after a pause, as though she'd had to force herself to pronounce it. "I do not want you to come in. I am not a masochist, and I do not want to be around anyone who makes me feel as badly as you make me feel. You made it clear how you feel about me. You said my whole life was a waste. You told me I was worthless and that you were ashamed to be my mother."

Until almost 1:00 A.M. I went over and over my responses to her repetitious erroneous charges. "I have never even thought those things, Ann. I have certainly been sorry that you have had so much trouble. There was never any question about loving you even in our worst of times. I only tried to tell you how I felt about the risks I thought you were taking with your health."

"That's right. You didn't want to be around anyone who wasn't healthy."

"Annie, hear me. I did not want you to be sick because your life has been meaningful to everyone in our family, and to your many, many friends. You are important to all of us."

"Really, Ma?" Every time I thought that she understood what I was saying, Ann began to recite the charges over again from the beginning as if she hadn't spoken. "I have to tell you, Ma. You said that I was worthless and that you are ashamed to be my mother. I cannot see you, Ma, unless you admit that you said those things."

Under different circumstances perhaps I would have given up, but this behavior on Ann's part connected with my deepest fear. I had worked with John Coffee, a young man who contracted AIDS through a blood transfusion. When he died I continued to see his wife in therapy. In helping them, I read everything I could find about AIDS. A recent study described the social withdrawal, mood disturbances, and memory abnormalities often present in persons suffering from the human immune deficiency virus, which sometimes infiltrated the brain long before the disease became diagnosable. The article banished any reassurance I felt in recalling that the nurses in the hospital had used no precautions, worn no rubber gloves, in administering Ann's transfusions. Frightened, I had called the Gay Men's Hot Line in New Haven for the name of a local doctor willing to treat AIDS. The anonymous man I spoke to talked about a Donald Evans, describing his rare compassion.

Now, regardless of our frustrating conversation, I wanted to get Ann to Dr. Evans.

"Annie," I said, "forgive me for whatever you think I might have said that hurt you. I just want to be able to help you until you're feeling better."

"But, Ma, you have to admit you said it. I cannot come home if you do not admit it. And can't you see that if you do, there is no way I can be with anyone who judges my whole life as being worthless? I don't want to hang up on you, but, good-bye, Ma."

May 1987

Mom, How can you possibly expect that I would
be able to share my shame with you who love me
and will feel pain at my defeat?
Not just momentary defeat.
I no longer have any hope
for myself, for my life.
But I am not cruel enough to inflict
that reality on others,
especially those I love.
And I am also not tough enough to maintain
the illusion that I'm OK
with people I love too well to lie to—
and love too well
NOT to lie to.
A dilemma. Stalemate.
Conclusion (by me) Withdrawal:
from the warmth and caring
that make life worthwhile.

ANN
(UNMAILED LETTER)

Together and Apart Again

For days I railed at the injustice of the position Ann had forced upon me. If I did not agree with her that I was ashamed to be her mother, we could not have a relationship. If I were to agree, we would not be able to connect because of my negative thoughts.

If she had been a patient, we might have found a way to break through her relentless opposition. The week I found Ann in the hospital I had seen a mother and daughter together in my office. It was the mother who said, "If that's the way you feel about me, get out of my life." But she was leaning toward the daughter as she spoke.

The thirty-four-year-old woman, exactly Ann's age, cried, "But that's just why I'm here. I feel as though I have never been in your life. I came here to change that."

I knew from Ann's condition that we might never have the time to sort through differences with a therapist. I had to find a way to reach her.

My dearest Ann,
I want to say, my dearest little girl—guess I'm getting like Grandpa was with me, not able to think of you and Rich and Bill

and Ellie as other than my children, regardless of the passage of time. Anyway, I want to say again how sorry I am about the misunderstandings you spoke about. I feel certain we can get beyond them.

Most important for now I want to tell you about a doctor in Newtown who has a reputation for his skill and empathy. Moreover, he is, I understand, well-versed in New York theater and art. His name is Dr. Evans. I think that you might like him. I would like to have you come home and make an appointment to see him.

For further incentive, Paul and I are going to New Hampshire on the weekend, to see Bill and Nicola. (It's hard for me to believe our Billy will be a father in November and that Ellie will be a mother for the second time only weeks after Nicola's due date.) We will be away from Saturday through Monday. If David could drive you out, you might enjoy the privacy (and rarity) of our house being quiet.

Then when I get home, in addition to my taking you to check out Dr. Evans, there's always Baskin-Robbins coffee ice cream sodas and rides out into the country, new cushions on the deck chairs and . . . Well, maybe you've figured it out—I'm trying to lure you home. PLEASE COME.

> I love you.
> Mom

My youngest stepson, Peter, stayed at our home the weekend Paul and I were in New Hampshire. Billy, both art and music critic for the regional paper, took us to a concert at Dartmouth. Nicola stayed home to frame some of her paintings for a show in Hanover. In their spare time they were fixing the sunroom for their baby.

We were at the kitchen table Sunday night, enjoying Billy's dill and carrot soup, when Peter called. David had driven Ann to the door. Her head and fingertips were bleeding. She went directly to bed. Peter brewed herb tea and brought it to her.

Paul and I left New Hampshire early in the morning and got home about eleven. I was stunned to find Tim Mitchell in the kitchen. "How did you know Ann was here?"

"I had no hope of running into Ann," Tim said. "I was up in Springfield visiting my parents and decided to stop by just to say hello to you and Paul. Ann was as surprised to see me as I was to find her here. She rushed upstairs to put something on her head. She seems to have some kind of wound."

Annie was in the bathroom trying to tie a scarf around her head. Her hands were shaking. "I can't believe that Tim showed up, Ma. I'm so upset to have him see me like this." She let me help with the scarf and wrap a Band-Aid around each of her bleeding fingertips. She needed to hold the railing to make her way down the stairs.

From my bedroom, I could see them on the deck. Ann was sitting in her favorite spot, close by the saltwater pond. I remembered when she and Tim chose to crowd into a single seat. Now their chairs were distant.

Soon they both stood up. They seemed to be saying a stilted good-bye.

Suddenly Tim reached out. He drew Ann to his chest, tenderly stroking her back. Before he left he kissed her cheeks and forehead. "Bye-bye, my Annadama," he called from the car.

Ann gave Tim the Irish Good-bye, waving with her eyes shut until his car was out of sight.

She slept most of Tuesday while Paul and I made the trip to Newtown to meet with Dr. Evans. I wanted to be certain we had found a doctor who would treat my wasted daughter with the dignity and respect we all wanted for her.

"He passes the first test," Paul said, picking up an Andy Warhol magazine in Dr. Evans's waiting room.

He came to greet us smiling, in a banana yellow jacket with an orchid-flowered tie. He nodded compassionately as Paul and I recited her medical history: Austen Riggs, Yale, two bouts of hepatitis, Silver Hill, biopsies, drug treatment programs.

"She's been through it all, hasn't she?" He shook his head. "And you, too, I imagine." His eyes searched mine.

"I'm afraid to hope that you can help her," I said. "We came to you knowing she has tested negative for AIDS in several hospitals in New York. Yet I cannot imagine what else would account for her condition. I'm afraid the tests were wrong and that she really does have a form of AIDS. Ann was in Africa eleven years ago. She was cut by witch doctors—"

Both Paul and Dr. Evans looked at me with a kind of silent concern. No, I was not denying her drug use. But she had suffered fevers of unknown origin episodically for eleven years. My step-son Peter, on his return from Africa, said AIDS was referred to there as "the thinness disease." Might it not be that all her years of thinness and debilitation had been caused by a strain of the virus that had yet to be detected by existing tests?

"I will not even venture to comment until I get to see her," the doctor said. He turned to his desk and wrote out a card. "Bring her here on Saturday at eleven. Till then, let's just keep on hoping that the tests in New York were correct."

"Do you really believe it all began in Africa?" Paul asked me, driving home.

"It would be easier to accept, somehow, if her problems began from a physical rather than a mental cause. Yet I would feel worse in one way, and that would be for blaming her for not taking care of herself when there was no way she really could, if she had AIDS that long."

"It's not an either/or situation," Paul said. "No matter what happened in Africa, she did abuse her body with drugs."

"I know."

All week Ann was feverish and exhausted. And yet I felt a sense of relief, almost exhilaration. I knew where she was. I could walk into the room and find her, touch her, speak to her.

On Saturday we went to Dr. Evans. He spoke cheerfully to Ann, but wanted us to go directly to the emergency room at the hospital. He would come to admit her.

Ann said she was not prepared. She had to gather up her books. She could not go to the hospital without them.

The doctor said, "Let your mother bring them later."

He saw that Ann was adamant. She would not go without returning home first. "Then I'll meet you at the hospital in an hour," he said.

I heard her calling David from her bedroom. "They're doing it again. Forcing me into a hospital. Come and get me, David."

I picked up the extension phone. "David, Dr. Evans is waiting. We both know that it's very hard for Ann to have to be admitted, but I'm sure you understand that she needs it. Why don't you meet us in the emergency room?"

"Get off the phone, please, Mother. I am speaking to my friend."

It was Paul who gently talked her into giving herself a chance to see if Dr. Evans could help. He carried her books to the car. It felt like one of those times with a little child when the dad could be more effective than the mother.

It was Memorial Day weekend. Sunshine. Parades. Picnics. Traffic crept along Route 7, thinning gradually until we reached the reservoir. I parked a few moments, hoping Ann would enjoy the cool deep blueness of the water, the lushness of the evergreens surrounding it.

She seemed to have forgotten our disagreement. "How beautiful, Mom. How lovely."

But at the hospital she refused to leave the car. "How would you feel, Mother, if you were giving up your freedom?" She crossed her arms and pressed her feet against the glove compartment.

"Awful, dear." I stood by her open door. "Unless I hoped it might be worth it. Then I'd try not to agonize. I'd just try to get started without too much thinking. I've brought you here because I'm praying that the pain you have been feeling will be alleviated."

I did have hope, if only that supervised administration of medications would relieve the thrush that led to body-racking coughing, relieve the leg cramps that caused her to cry out at night, reduce the raging fevers.

Finally, Annie stopped resisting and let me take her hand. She put one foot and then another onto the blacktop. She collapsed at the door to the emergency entrance. An orderly came running with a wheelchair.

I got my wish the first week. Ann's symptoms were relieved.

The thrush and leg cramps were under control. She was feeling better. But the second week her X rays indicated the likelihood of TB. Ann was wheeled down the hall to a pressure-treated room, where breathing would be easier. It took her just a minute to comment that the new room overlooked a cemetery.

Fevers spiked and lowered unpredictably. The outer door to her room was plastered with blue, red, and yellow precautions. Blood, urine, smoking, infectious disease warnings. Paul, David, and I were instructed to put on hospital gowns, masks, and rubber gloves before we went to see her, and to scrub with surgical soap on departing. Still we had no final diagnosis.

The kindly nurses said the Western Blot Test took ten days to two weeks to determine Acquired Immune Deficiency. Dr. Evans was presenting a paper at the first International Conference on AIDS, in Washington, D.C. I wondered whether test results were being held until he himself could tell us.

I was with her the day he returned. Ann smiled at him. She could not remember his name. She solved the problem by renaming the doctor after her favorite brand of ice cream.

"Well, look who's here, Ma. It's Dr. Baskin-Robbins!"

The doctor reached out for her hand.

"I'm glad you came back," she said, and then her expression changed. "I don't seem able to make any sense of myself. I find it very frightening. But first, how was the conference?"

"Very interesting. Say, who are all these folks?" He studied the cork board where I had taped photographs of friends and family. It felt as though both Ann and Dr. Evans were engaged in some mutual avoidance dance.

Ann had a tale to tell with every picture. He stood and nodded through the lengthy presentation. Finally he turned to me. "May I speak to Annie alone? I'll meet you in the waiting room."

While Dr. Evans spoke to Ann I went to the little chapel and knelt before the stained-glass window. O, please God, whatever Ann and I have to hear tonight—give us the strength to bear it, I thought.

I knew by his face the news he must have told her. "Then Ann really does have AIDS?" I knew but spoke it like a question.

"Of course." He nodded, cupping his hand under my elbow as though he thought that I might fall.

"And you told her?"

"Of course." He nodded.

"How long would you think she can live?"

"She'll make it through the summer," he said slowly. "I don't expect she'll be around for Christmas."

I heard the words. I could not accept their meaning. Although I had been haunted by the thought of AIDS, this confirmation provoked an overwhelming feeling of denial.

"Well, see you tomorrow. Try to take care of yourself." Dr. Evans turned to leave. I saw that he had tears in his eyes.

I sobbed in the ladies' room, then wiped my face with a wet paper towel. Trembling, I put on the paper gown and rubber gloves and went to my daughter's bedside.

Ann was sitting up, knees drawn to her chest like a child. She reached for my hand. "Mamma—do you think it might not even be true? I took a lot of tests in New York. Every one was negative. How am I supposed to know? How are you supposed to know? I never tested positive before. It might be something being done to me." She bit her lip. Her eyes pleaded with mine.

The tears started down my cheeks. Then she cried too.

"Promise one thing, Mamma. When I get out of here we'll go for one more test. Some other place."

"I promise." I squeezed her hand. "And whatever we have to face, you promise me that we'll do it together. No more disappearing, Annie."

"I promise."

She wanted me to write to Randy. I was not to tell him her condition. She said she had to know if he was well. "Randy is the only one I ever did heroin with. If he is okay, then I cannot believe that I have AIDS."

His response arrived within a week. Ann asked me to read it to her several times.

"Oh, Ma," she smiled, "it sounds exactly like Randy."

Eleanor,

8am in the guest house in hollywood. It made me so happy to get your note. I'd been meaning to get in touch. I used you as a reference for a few job possibilities and i trust you will tell anyone who asks that Randy Slade and your daughter were drug addicts together. Bad joke. Hey, but i got a real cool gig. I drive thru the vast system of arteries radaring my way in a sea of traffic they call L.A. I'm working for a courier service who deals mainly with the studios raydio and mass media in general, so i get to drive to all sorts of interesting places. god, it's 10 to 6 mon to fri—i feel so normal: It's truly the very thing i was looking for 2oo cash a week and nobody breathing down my back. Hope to sail it right thru the summer. But of course somewhere deep theres this burning desire to rock n roll. The child who needs to fly. Conjour the pure spirit for i'm living in the city of light. But i ain't losin my head no more for if theres anything i'm learnin thats how to be free. Guess it takes work to be free. The lightness is no longer unbearable. I feel like a man on a tightrope, we must conquer our fear of falling. Eleanor, it's so good to be speaking with you. There's so much information we could share. I remember you saying once you didnt know what it meant to pray. Well, It's a subject i have pondered, so im enclosing a little diddy which attempts to confront the issue. Ann is, or thinks she is, an authority on this matter. I shudder to think of all the candles and nameless saints. And yet to meet one so intensely religious, who takes life so seriously. Oh to start conjuring ann up is yes painful. For when i think of the potential, and all our shattered dreams, i just feel so helpless. You said she has not been well. So i send out this prayer:

> *may she the holy spirit*
> *find it's way into her soul*
> *and heal, bless and release her*
> *and her spirit shall soar.*

So anyway, i'm gonna jump in the shower and get clean. I love you Eleanor, let's stay in touch.

Randy

That night Ann called Randy and told him she had AIDS.

I have brought myself
to fairly bitter circumstances.
Fiercely painful, yes;
and of course my own fault.
Each day, each minute I discover
how very much more damaged I am
than I have been willing to acknowledge.
Paralyzing the shame,
the denial,
the relentless regret.

(DIARY ENTRY, JUNE 1987)

But Ann was not yet able to confront the truth with her family. On June 18 she dictated a birthday note for me to send her father assuring him that she was doing well.

Dearest Pop,
I love you and hope you have a terrific birthday.
   I am doing great, I know you'll be thrilled to know.
                              Love,
                              Ann.

While notes she wrote to herself conveyed the depth of her despair:

My circumstance:
Physical: Menopause?
Muscle shrinkage to point of no return,
loss of pubic hair and body hair, loss of
head hair, swallowing problems, rash,
thrush,
Fucking aids?
teeth—dead teeth must be removed (only six teeth left!)
Social: What the fuck is my life
   (Answer) Blown
Drink too much because I am so scared to face my reality.
Utterly horrified by what I have done

> *(to myself, to everyone around me),*
> *I have devastated myself—blasted*
> *every potential aspect of myself out*
> *of existence and left*
> *myself without a past, a present*
> *or possibly a future.*
> *how horrifying to find*
> *yourself a living B movie cliché*
> *the "has been"*
> *no, more precisely*
> *the "almost-was"*

(DIARY ENTRY, JULY 1987)

Dr. Evans saw her bouts of depression. "I think I know what would help. How would you like to go out for a pass?"

"Well . . ." Ann cast her eyes down on the lines of tubing connected into the shunt that had been surgically implanted into her chest. "I can't believe that I would say I'd rather sit here in this nice hospital. Hospital! I can't believe it. . . ."

"Don't be afraid." He sat on the edge of her bed. "You don't have to stay connected to these tubes all the time. Your own batteries will work just fine. We can unhook you a few hours at a time any afternoon or evening you feel ready. I'll leave a standing order with the nurses."

"It's not that I'm afraid, Ma," she told me. "It's that I look so awful. No teeth. No hair."

I found her fancy turbans. Dr. Evans ordered her to be wheeled over to the dental lab.

The beautiful plastic teeth restored a look of fragile glamour. Ann scrawled a heartfelt note to the dentist:

> So, Dr. Hinden, thanks for your kindness. I was very frightened that you'd snigger and perhaps vomit when you took a look. Instead you mentioned that a mouth like mine probably HURT, which made me feel better. Lots better!

David was the first to take her out. She returned to the hospital radiant.

Then it was to be my turn. We were going to the closest Baskin-Robbins. But before I finished seeing clients, Ann had left a message on the answering machine at my office.

"Ma, my great new teeth are broken. I let them sit in a glass on my table. When I looked again they were on the floor, split into little pieces. I cannot for the life of me figure out what happened. What am I supposed to do now? I don't want to go out. I feel so confused by everything."

Dr. Hinden fixed her teeth again. Either David or I took Ann out every other day. I became an expert at returning the stares that Ann's appearance engendered. I even went up to people in stores and said:

It isn't kind to stare. . . .

She is not well. . . .

Can you be compassionate. . . .

If she were someone you loved. . . .

Then Ann's outings had to be postponed because of raging fevers, insatiable fatigue, sad episodes of dementia. Once when she seemed to be sleeping, Annie kept repeating in a kind of gospel singsong "Ooo, ooo child, things are gonna be easier. . . ." Quickly, and yet each time more briefly, powerful intravenous drugs and two or three transfusions of blood brought Ann back from hallucinating.

> *You can no longer determine boundaries*
> *between one dimension and another*
> *Vibrations of sound*
> *of light of flesh of matter of pain*
> *vibrations of thought of time*
> *all dance as one*
>
> (DIARY ENTRY, AUGUST 1987)

One danger in being close to Ann at times was that some opportunistic diseases that may set in with AIDS are contagious. When Ann was being checked for TB and for viral pneumonia, I had to wear a face mask. Ellen, whose pregnancy made her more vulnerable to infection, was not allowed to visit at all until Ann had been in the hospital almost two months and was in relatively stable condition.

Ann was very excited about Ellen's visit and begged permission for little Charlie to come as well. Dr. Evans not only agreed but urged us to have a family picnic out on the doctors' patio. Two-and-a-half-year-old Charlie insisted on pushing Annie's wheel-chair around the patio. Ellie and I let ourselves bask in the August sunshine. We said very little. It was enough just to be together.

Charlie halted the wheelchair. "Look, Annie," he said, point-ing to a bird in flight. "See that bird? That's my bird. That bird is named Charlie like I am."

Ann smiled. "Hellooo, Charlie Bird! I wish I had a bird too. Charlie Bird is beautiful."

Annie got chilled easily. As the shadows lengthened Ellen vol-unteered to wheel her sister back to her hospital room. They would have a chance to be alone. I held Charlie's hand and we walked toward the outside stairway.

"Wait, Bamma!" Charlie suddenly broke away from me and ran toward Annie and his mother. "Annie! Guess what? I just saw a Annie Bird up in the sky with my Charlie Bird!"

From somewhere down a hallway Ann's voice came echoing back. "Charlie, Charlie, thank you! Tell my bird to keep on flying!"

Ann began to talk about each of the children in the family. She wrote to Richard's five-year-old:

> From: Ann To: Zoya
> How is my dear little Zoya?
> I loved my card from you. It made me feel so much better. Tell me about Hong Kong. I bet you're a little bit lonely, but just wait. Another couple months and you'll never want to come home.
> What is your apartment like? Or is it a house? I hear your Daddy is going on a trip pretty soon. Maybe we will get to see him and he will tell us all about you. And about little David too. Is he growing up?

Well my very dear little girl, my Zoya, I love you so much you won't believe it.

Please remember that always.

Ann

Ann had been in the hospital for a month when Richard, by extending a business trip to Europe, was able to arrange the time to visit. Dr. Evans allowed an all-day pass, beginning with our taking her out for breakfast.

Ann was thrilled to see her brother. Looking radiant in a white turban and white jumpsuit, she was waiting in the hallway in a wheelchair when Richard and I stepped out of the elevator.

Tall, handsome Richie opened his strong arms and ran to embrace his sister. "Annie, Annie," Richard said. Their hug was long and silent.

When he stepped back, she looked at him the way she used to "check him out" before he went on dates.

"Clearly the man is a rising star!" Then Ann made motor noises. "Varoom, varoom, get me outta here, Bro!"

We stopped at Friendly's for breakfast. I was planning to bring the food to the car, but Ann felt strong enough to walk into the restaurant. We sat about an hour in a corner booth while Rich told stories about Hong Kong, the view of the harbor from their apartment, how Zoya and David loved taking the Star Ferry to Kowloon, Rosemary's incredible initiative in finding a job as psychologist at the International School within days of their arrival, his own work managing trade shows in Shanghai and Beijing.

"I'm so proud of you, Rich." Ann put her hand on his. I was glad she was not bleeding, glad that Rich was with her on a good day.

Driving through the countryside, Ann asked to stop at a roadside farm store stocked with fruits, vegetables, homemade pies, jams, and jellies. I was paying for the apple-cranberry jelly she wanted to bring back to the nurses when a blister that had not been apparent underneath her lipstick suddenly burst, dripping blood down her chin and onto her white sweater.

Rich and I looked at one another in distress. Wiping her mouth,

Ann got blood on her hand. It was terrifying to know that the fluid was deadly. We had to get her out of there before she touched any food.

"What happened to you?" the white-haired woman proprietor stared.

Before I could think of how to rescue her, Ann answered in a friendly way. "Got hit in the mouth in a baseball game this morning."

"That so?" The woman's eyes narrowed. "Awfully early t'be playin' baseball."

"Yup, awful early," Ann repeated, dabbing at her mouth again. "But the good news is we won the game."

"Well, see you later now." Rich and I headed for the car, grateful that Ann, who liked to linger, decided to follow.

"Quick, Rich." I pulled four plastic gloves from my purse.

He looked upset. "Won't Annie be hurt?"

I realized he had not been exposed to the self-protective measures we who saw her often had become accustomed to now.

"There isn't any choice, Rich."

Ann entered the car, and winced at the gloved hand with which I handed her a pack of tissues.

I drove further into the countryside, intent on avoiding any possible contact with people. An hour later we happened on a lovely lake rimmed by giant pine trees. Rich and I sat on big rocks to watch Ann wade.

"Oh, this feels so great!" Cupping the water, she washed her face and arms. "Look, Rich." She bent and squinted to see through the water. "I found a heart-shaped stone for Zoya. And here's a good-luck one with a ring around it for David." Annie dropped the stones in her brother's gloved hand.

We basked together in the sun. For a while, just being with Richie and Ann, listening to their stories of how they turned the chicken coop into a clubhouse, played king-of-the-mountain on sand drifts, had a secret language no other kids could understand, I felt almost relaxed enough to forget her condition. Then I saw that Annie's lip had begun to drip again. I stood up and said we'd better think about returning to the hospital.

Ann fell asleep on the way back. She woke as Richard brought the wheelchair to the car.

In her room, ensconced on her pillows, Ann's vitality returned. "Our man in Hong Kong," she grinned at her brother. Then her expression changed. "Rich," she said, "before you leave there is something I have to tell you."

Richard sat on his sister's bed. She put her hand on his rubber-gloved palm.

"I have a sort of embarrassing thing going on. I have a kind of gastrointestinal thrush that needs a lot of monitoring. I keep taking a lot of medications, but nothing is helping enough. They say I have a kind of immune deficiency, Rich, and that leaves me wide open to any infection. My body cannot even fight the thrush in my throat. It's gone down to my lungs."

"Annie," Richard swallowed hard, "does it hurt?"

"Not as much as the mental pain." She shook her head and looked toward the window. "So hope and pray, eh, Bro? I really wanted to see Zoya and David grow up."

"I always tell them about things we did when we were their ages." Richie's voice cracked. "Remember playing ghost, and dressing Ellie up as the New Year's baby? And remember the crazy cereal cookies you used to make us for breakfast?"

"Peanut butter mixed with Cheerios?" Ann tried to sound indignant. "What's so crazy about that!" Then she stroked Richard's black hair. "We did have lots of fun as kids together, didn't we, Rich? I have so many happy memories."

At four o'clock she began to fall asleep again.

"Good-bye, Annie." Richie bent to kiss her forehead. She did not open her eyes until he tiptoed out the door.

"Richard!" she called, waking as if startled. "Please come back a moment!"

Annie wagged her bandaged finger at her younger brother. "I have one more thing I want you to remember, and that is always—always—I want you to keep fun in your heart!"

Richard and I stopped at the reservoir and cried together. Then we laughed through our tears as Richie recalled her quick response to the woman in the farm shop.

Richard sent a card on his return to Hong Kong. Ann was unable to read it.

"Periodic bleeding in the retina," Dr. Evans explained.

"Who is that?" she would ask, pointing to a picture of one of her brothers or of Tim or David. She began to print in capital letters, using a thick black marker. One afternoon I found a note in her room:

DEAREST MOM—STAY HERE PLEASE. I SHOULD BE BACK IN HALF AN HOUR FROM NOW WHICH IS QUARTER OF—OR SOMETHING PAST?
LOVE, ANN

I waited half an hour, then went to look for her in the laboratories where she might have been sent for testing. I found her slumped in her wheelchair in the waiting area for CAT scans. "I'm all through here, Ma, but no one seemed to want to push my wheelchair. They said for me to wait for a volunteer or someone."

"We don't have to wait for anyone, Annie. In fact this tour will stop at the coffee shop for take-out ice cream sodas."

In spite of the disappointments and setbacks I sometimes felt a kind of comfort. I did not have to wake at night wondering whether Ann was on the streets of the Lower East Side. She slept on clean sheets. The care she got was splendid, the nurses kind and patient. She was sick, but I could be with her, and she was not alone.

In mid-August, Paul and I drove up to Boston. Over a year had passed since his mother's death. For the first time since her funeral her three children could be together to honor the memory of this strong woman by unveiling the monument to her at a cemetery near Boston.

Paul's brother Norman and his wife, Pat, had flown in from London. His sister Pat and brother-in-law Saul were coming in from Florida.

We met the family at the cemetery at noontime. The ceremony

was brief but touching. Each of Bertha's three middle-aged children remembered special incidents: her journey to America from Russia alone at the age of sixteen, how the young Boston doctor had fallen in love with the beautiful immigrant. Her surviving brother Henry wept as he remembered his older sister. Thirty-two others in their family, their father included, had died at death camps in Poland.

We had the use of a relative's apartment in Cambridge, overlooking a bend in the Charles River, for a family gathering following the service. We were still at the table lingering over coffee and memories of Bertha when the telephone rang.

"Hello, my name is Gerry. I'm not the regular nurse, just substituting today on Ten West. I tried to get you at home. Your son gave me this number. I think you ought to know that Ann Craig is in poor condition and may not last through the evening."

Paul sped me to the hospital. On the three-hour drive from Boston to Danbury I told him what the nurse had said; Dr. Evans had ordered a two-unit blood transfusion to boost Ann's depleted white cell count. She had fallen asleep during the transfusion. The nurse named Gerry had tiptoed into the room and raised the bed rails so she would neither fall nor try to get up while blood was being administered. Ann woke to the darkened room, somehow reached a pair of scissors, and cut the tubing to free herself. Sometime later the nurse had found her semiconscious on the floor. She had lost a third of her own blood.

> I think of strange things swollen
> purple rills of flesh spitting
> fire and lightning
> I realize with a start that
> I am badly in need of air or
> that I have not breathed out or
> taken breath in for far too long a time
> that indeed my lungs have been pained
> my body tensed and I have not
> noticed attention focused elsewhere

> *attention sucked*
> *into some concerting train of thought*
>   (DIARY ENTRY, AUGUST 1987)

We pulled into the parking garage next to the hospital at about
7:30. As we reached the elevator I saw that Paul's hand trembled
as he reached to press the up button. In the tenth-floor anteroom
we helped each other tie on surgical masks and don the yellow
paper gowns and familiar rubber gloves.

I prayed I would have the courage to accept the worst. I opened
the door to my daughter's room.

Ann was sitting up in bed, two pillows propped behind her.
Three lines of intravenous fluid, two clear and one red, led to the
shunt in her chest.

"Oh, no!" she turned to the nurse beside her. "Don't tell me
you called my mother. Mom. Paul. I am so embarrassed! It was
such a stupid thing to do. I woke up all confused and not remembering that I was in the hospital. I thought I was having some
kind of nightmare and that I was caught in a cage. I had no
memory of the nurse pulling up the bed rails. All I knew was that
I had to get out. I can't believe they called you up over such a
nutty incident."

"I'm calling her the miracle kid." The gray-haired nurse stood
shaking her head. "I never saw anyone rally so quickly to intravenous fluids."

Soon Paul was telling Ann ideas about his latest venture, a
magazine for active adults. I was grateful to him for so quickly
shifting the focus away from her condition.

"Sounds great, Paul," she grinned. "How 'bout I write the travel
column? You could send me to Tahiti or Morocco. Or maybe we
should start with Nairobi?"

On the way home I put my hand over Paul's. "I'm sorry," I
said. "You couldn't even have the memorial service for your
mother without a crisis with Ann."

"I love her, too," he said. "Don't you forget it."

Ann slept more often after that. About a week later she asked
if I knew how to get in touch with Tim.

I called and Tim drove out from New York to the hospital the following afternoon.

"Oh no, Ma. Don't let him see me," Ann cried when the nurse announced that he was waiting in the hallway. "I look awful today. It's the worst time he could have chosen."

It took half an hour for me to help her tie the flowered turban about her bandaged head, and exchange the hospital gown for her rose-colored jacket and black silk slacks. Then, holding on to the bed, the walls, the railings in the bathroom, she made her way to the mirror to layer the thick black stage makeup around her eyes.

Finally, propped up in her bed, Ann called, "I heard there's a real cute fellow out in the hall. Would he like to come in?"

"Annadama." Tim, rubber-gloved and tied into a yellow gown, came through the door with his arms extended. His voice was muffled through the surgical mask.

"Thanks for letting me visit." He pulled off the mask and gloves and went directly to embrace her.

"I'll see you two later." I started to leave the room.

"Oh no, Ma, please finish fixing the flowers. When the flowers die," Ann turned to Tim, "my mother keeps replacing them with silk ones. She brought these pink ones today. Would you put them in that basket where those roses died, Ma?" Ann pointed. "But save the rose petals for me. You know I like to smell them."

While I arranged the flowers, Tim presented Ann with two brown paper bags secured with rubber bands.

"Definitely the male touch on the gift wrap, Tim," she laughed. "Oh, exactly what I need here." The first bag contained a small black boxing glove connected to a hinged device. "So you can punch out anyone who tries to hurt you, Annadama," Tim said. His second gift was a plastic crocodile head with hinged mouth mounted on a rod enabling the holder to pick up books and papers in the serpent's jaws.

"Not that I think anything could be beyond your own reach, Tootsie." Tim smiled as Ann, with ferocious noises, made the crocodile snap at his nose.

I fussed with flowers while they talked about the screenplay

Tim was writing. Ann's voice began to fade. She sank back into her pillow with her eyes closed. Tim and I looked at her and then at each other. We waited several minutes.

"Tim," she said softly, "please hold my hand. The doctor said I am going to die. What do you think will happen to me? I'm frightened."

"Oh, Tootsie," Tim held on to her right hand. "My Tootsie," he paused, "the fear will come and the fear will go. Don't you remember how scared we were about going to Africa? And how wonderful it all turned out to be? Well," with his left hand Tim stroked her trembling face, "I think it will be an adventure—even more mysterious, more beautiful than Africa."

I tiptoed out of the room.

Tim and I met for dinner at a seafood restaurant in downtown Danbury. He spoke lovingly about the first time he saw Ann. "I was shooting a film from a rooftop in Providence. Suddenly I spotted this glorious-looking girl across the street. I swear to you I almost fell off that roof. I told her I could get her into movies. She said I ought to find a writer who could feed me better lines."

We laughed and then fell silent.

"Tell me, please," Tim finally spoke again. "Has the doctor said how long she might go on?"

"A few months at best."

"Oh, my beautiful Annie." Tim sucked in his breath and closed his eyes. "I am so very sorry. And sorry for her mamma." He looked at me. "You two have such a bond. It must have been a terrible blow to hear the diagnosis."

"Tim, for the past few years my greatest fear was finding out that Annie had died alone in the city. Is it possible to understand that I am strangely grateful that this horrible disease allows her family to be with her when it's time to say good-bye?"

"This afternoon," Tim said softly, "she asked me to come back with something from our travels that she could hold on to for comfort and for courage. Then she asked if I could remember the message we found scratched on a wall at an old African seaport, from which slaves had been shipped to Europe. They were the last words the poor people saw as they were wrenched from their families. Annie said them after me today:

> "Here leave the memory of your loved one.
> Lay down the burden of your heart."

Over coffee, Tim said, "Did it seem to you that Ann went through a personality change after the rape in Germany?"

My silence must have caused him to look up. Tim rightly judged that I had never known she had been raped. "Forgive me," he said. "What an awful time to tell you."

At first I couldn't talk. "God, it hurts. Why wouldn't she have told me? Why couldn't I have helped her?"

"I'm sure she didn't want to hurt you. I also remember her saying she thought that if she made it public it would put an end to her father's research in Germany. I know at the time only her friend Eric knew, and she swore him to secrecy. But I always thought of that night as the turning point that robbed Ann of her self-esteem."

Haltingly at first, Tim recounted what Ann told him. As he spoke, I remembered my own version of the evening.

It had all begun so happily, packing up our family to spend a year in Germany while Bill was doing research. The four children entered the Frankfurt International School and Ann was soon experiencing her first romance. With their blue eyes, mahogany hair, and freckles, Ann and Eric looked like brother and sister. She was sixteen years old.

> Loving you has been an experience, Eric said, propping up his elbow on a small fluffy cloud. In what manner, I replied, brushing the stardust out of my hair.
>
> (DIARY ENTRY, JANUARY 1969)

On May 23, she was to attend Eric's graduation party. It was a balmy evening and our family ate supper on the little balcony of our apartment, from which we watched the sun set beyond the

Taunus Mountains. As the radiance faded a crescent moon appeared.

Annie left the darkened balcony to dress for Eric's party. Billy, Ellen, and I walked to the end of the block to get the car so I could drive her. But it was not where I had parked it. We continued looking, unable to believe our Opal had been stolen.

Bill phoned the police. We disagreed about sending her off by taxi. I wanted her to be able to go regardless of the missing car. She and Eric would say good-bye in just a few more days, he to return to Canada with his family.

Waiting for the taxi, I braided a pale pink satin ribbon into Annie's curly hair. She looked like a junior Katharine Hepburn, her high cheekbones and deep-set eyes shining with excitement.

"Let me know who's driving you home." I hugged her as the driver honked outside our apartment.

"Don't worry, Ma," she rushed down the stairs. "I'll call you later."

But she didn't.

It was close to midnight when her classmate's father brought Ann home, all color drained from her face, her body wracked with shudders. The palm of her hand was so severely burned that Bill rushed her to the military hospital for treatment. She told us she had placed her hand on a stovepipe.

I had to pull away from my own remembrances to pay attention to what Tim was saying.

The class of 1969 decided to meet at someone's home, rather than at the inn in Oberursal. Not knowing the locale was changed, Ann waited at the inn for her friends. Eric drove to get her. But distances were long. The bartender, whose name was Wilfred, began a conversation. Suddenly he held her hand on a stovepipe until she was too pained to resist his sexual assault.

> When I could no longer fight you
> I left my body and was dead
> The little girl whose body you were violating
> Watched down on you from the ceiling.

What you did, you did to her dead body
—no right to life—entitled only to a dead life.
Being dead—you cannot kill me.

I had to die to keep from dying
Not from your cruelty—
But from my feelings.

I told them I had burned my hand
I did not say a child had been murdered.—

(DIARY ENTRY, MAY 24, 1969)

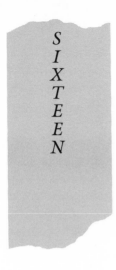

Who Is J?

Three days later Ann had another hard day and evening. I stayed by her bed, watching and hoping as a new medication dripped into her body. She lay white and motionless, tucked under the stiff hospital sheet. Several times an hour she would thrash and murmur phrases I could not always hear: "She wanted to die as John Doe. She did not want to hurt them." Then she began repeating words used to introduce a network radio news program. "You give me twenty-two minutes and I'll give you the world."

I brought her supper tray in from the hallway, propped her pillows, and tried to feed her sips of chicken consommé.

"I'm sorry, Ma." Ann shook her head when I raised the spoon. "I feel groggy beyond belief. I—I keep on seeing things and I never know what I'm looking at. People who were supposed to be dead but didn't quite die until they had imparted their secrets."

"What were their secrets, Annie dear?"

"That's just it, Ma. I—I don't know yet." She sank down into her pillow. "Unh—roses, please," she murmured. "Unh—roses, please."

Late that night, I bent to kiss her fevered forehead. Even as she slept, the television continued softly. I did not turn it off. She liked to waken to the sound of it. Tiptoeing from the room, I paused to hear the lead news item:

"Good evening. We begin the 'News at Eleven' with a worrisome statistic. AIDS is killing more women in the twenty-six to thirty-five-year age group in New York City than cancer. Eighty percent of those infected have been intravenous drug users. . . ."

In the anteroom, I peeled off the rubber gloves and took a long time scrubbing my hands and face with the green pine-scented liquid soap.

On the long drive home I heard myself singing, over and over again:

> Go to sleep my little baby
> Or the boogyman will get you
> When you wake
> You may have a piece of cake. . . .

Paul was already asleep by the time I got home at one. Restless, I laid awake, envisioning Ann with all the tubes going into her chest, perhaps awake now and all alone in the isolated room, having night sweats.

Trying to distract myself, I tuned into the radio softly enough not to bother Paul, and stayed awake through a talk show interview with a man who told about being held in captivity, undergoing detailed physical examination at the mercy of creatures from another planet. News. Music. A female psychologist doing instant therapy with phone-in clients. More news. More music until sleep finally came, as it will, just an hour before I had to get up.

I woke to both Paul's singing in the shower and the radio playing directly by my head. It took a minute for me to realize that AIDS was the topic of discussion.

". . . that this woman," the host was ranting, "a woman who is known to have AIDS, this woman who lives on an Army base, wife of a sergeant in the United States Army, this knowingly promiscuous woman is probably right at this moment spreading disease to some young American boy who is on that base in the service of our country! And I say we have to give authorities the right to lock her up. Lock her up and throw away the key! For-ever . . . !"

"Paul, can you hear this guy?" I yelled, but the shower was still running and apparently he could not hear me either.

"Time is running out, folks," the announcer kept raging. "Either speak out now or understand that you are going to be a victim of every homosexual, every junky-addict, and all the other scum who threaten to bring this nation to a halt. AIDS, friends. What do you think we should do to stop these people, those menaces to us, to our children, and to our country? What about this woman on the Army base? Let me hear what you think, huh? Remember, just dial seven-four-seven-WRBA. . . ."

With fierce determination, I instantly grabbed the telephone. I could not confront whoever the God was who was taking away my daughter, but I could, on her behalf, fight every fight that she would have to leave unfinished.

It rang a dozen times before a woman answered. "WRBA. Do you have something to say to Terry Becker?"

"I do. My daughter is in the hospital now, critically ill with AIDS. And I am infuriated by his sensationalistic approach to the subject."

"Hold on—" She cut me off. "I'll put you on the air right after the next commercial."

"Paul." He was heading from shower to closet, wrapped in a big blue towel. "Paul, take the radio out into the hall and listen! I'm about to be interviewed on WRBA."

He looked at me dubiously, but left the room with the radio under his arm.

"Terry Becker here. To whom am I speaking?"

"My name is Eleanor, and Mr. Becker, you are doing a cruel disservice to people who are suffering terribly. Have you ever seen what happens to people with AIDS? My daughter is in the hospital right now, like so many others, bleeding internally, having trouble breathing, too weak to walk—and you are sensationalizing one single situation."

"That's unfortunate about your daughter, Eleanor, but what

do you think should be done with a woman on an Army base deliberately spreading AIDS to our soldiers?"

"Where is the doctor who rendered that diagnosis? And what about her husband?" I had no idea what I was going to say, the words tumbled out before I consciously thought them. "If she is emotionally unstable, it is their responsibility to protect her from herself, and in so doing, they protect the others. Perhaps the woman you refer to has been neurologically impaired by the virus."

"We are almost out of time, Eleanor, but before we go, I have one other question for you. Just—how—" he emphasized each word. "Exactly—how—did—your—daughter—get—this disease? How did your daughter get AIDS, Eleanor?"

I heard his effort to discredit me. But most of all, to discredit Ann. I heard myself begin to stumble. "Probably, most probably, from a needle." Then the words began to flow again. "Perhaps even from extensive travel in Africa. Does it really matter, Mr. Becker? Do you suggest we blame the victims? This disease is a terrible tragedy, and no one deserves the suffering it engenders. We all must let it enhance our capacity for compassion."

A phrase of music indicated that the show was over. "Terry Becker here, for WRBA. Tomorrow, I'll be asking what you think of those nuns, throwing blood on the electric boat up there in Groton, Connecticut. Right now, stay tuned for the eight o'clock news."

Paul came in from the hallway, radio tucked under his arm, both hands gesturing thumbs up to me. "I can't believe you," he said. Paul had tears in his eyes. I sat on the side of my bed, clutching him, trembling, as he hugged me.

I couldn't wait to tell Annie. Couldn't wait to tell her that I spoke up for her and for all the people with AIDS. I would bring breakfast for both of us; French toast with real maple syrup, a change from the routine hospital food.

As I got into the protective paper gown and rubber gloves I sang through the door to Annie:

"Wake up! Wake up! You great big sleepy head."

And she sang back the response from her childhood, "All right. All right. I'll jump right out of bed."

Annie was thrilled by my story. We had a wonderful breakfast together, both of us sitting in chairs, me in the yellow hospital gown, Annie in her white robe and matching turban. We lined up two tray stands to make a table between us. The pleasure of the hot coffee and fresh orange juice was interrupted only by Ann repeating the story to every person who entered her room.

"Do you know what my mom did this morning?" she asked John, the custodian, as he emptied the wastebasket; Kathy, her pretty blond nurse; the unexpressive lab technician who came to draw blood samples. By the time Dr. Evans was making his rounds, the tale had grown to me being interviewed on national radio, telling everyone in America about my daughter's struggle and how we all had to rally together to find a cure for AIDS.

The following morning I got up early for a 7:30 appointment with a couple I had been seeing for about three months. I waited at the office with a mounting sense of agitation, not because they were late, but because I began to hope they would not arrive.

Yesterday's breakfast with Annie was such a special event, I wanted to repeat it. She seemed better, more alert in the morning. I did not want to miss the chance to be with her.

I left a hurried note for my would-be clients: "Sorry we did not connect this morning. Please call to reschedule," and headed for my car. Even pulling away I was afraid they might drive in and I would have to honor their appointment.

I sped to the hospital, then found myself walking into the gift shop to browse, rather than heading for the bank of elevators. What was I avoiding? That today would be a let-down after yesterday? That was silly, I chastised myself. Ann did not need to be "up" for my sake.

Approaching her corner room, last door on the right at the end of the hall, I could see that once again her tray had been left outside, a recurring problem each time a new kitchen aide saw the pink, yellow, and blue precaution signs taped to her outer door. The nurses were kind but too preoccupied with the urgent needs of pre- and postsurgical patients to notice a single meal left undelivered.

I lifted the cover. Her eggs were as cold as the metal tray. I would see that Annie had an appetizing breakfast.

One of the nurse's aides followed me to the tiny kitchen and stood between me and the microwave oven.

"Has that food been in Ann's room?" she pointed accusingly.

"I wish it had," I said. "I wouldn't be warming it up if someone had brought it to Ann." I stepped around her and set the timer on the microwave.

But I halted at the doorway, frozen with fear at the sight of Annie's face covered by her sheet. I watched to see if the sheet moved. Held my breath waiting to see if she were breathing.

The part of the sheet that covered her chest rose almost imperceptibly. I had to see it happen twice before I could be sure. Then I tiptoed to her side to uncover her face. She was sweating profusely. As I wiped her with a dampened facecloth, Ann began to waken.

"Mamma," she blinked. "Did we—or uh did we not—just watch a movie? A—about someone being kidnapped. We guess she is alive, but who can really say. Who has final authority?"

She looked toward the window as though she were watching TV. Her lips formed words of silent conversation.

"Let me feed you, darling." I brought the tray to her bedside but Annie showed no interest.

"I keep having this dream, Mom, that I am J. I cannot figure it out. What is the J?" She spoke hesitantly, her eyes still fixed on the window. "Do you think it means that—that I am Jesus? I know it does not mean that I am Jesus in the leadership way."

"Oh, Annie," I sat on the bed beside her, my arm light on her fragile shoulders, "I think the J means the spirit of Jesus is with you. The spirit that promises us love and peace and eternal life."

"That's what I thought it meant." Annie closed her eyes and slept the rest of the morning.

A Swim
for Annie

Saturday morning I did not attempt to bring breakfast to Annie at the hospital again. Instead I got to the beach before weekend sun worshipers were even out of bed. I wanted to be able to sit exactly where Ann liked to sit, in front of the pavilion on the firm sand close to the water. Except for an occasional jogger, the sea gulls and I laid claim to the vast expanse of seashore.

To my left, like a giant's finger, the rocky jetty pointed directly to the patch of scarlet sky now heralding the sun's arrival. I stood waist-deep in the chilly water watching the rising sun unfurl a golden pathway from the far horizon across the ocean's surface directly to my body.

This is for you, my Annie. If you are never going to swim again, every time I swim, I will swim for you. Tears hot on my face, I plunged into the sun-split sea and swam until I was exhausted.

> I am alone on the beach
> with the gulls
> the silent sleeping snails
> and the darting fish
> Alone with all of life
> stretched out before me.

Eleanor Craig

Silverfish patter
at my toes
I wade through
the dawn-pinked water
The golden sun
staining the sea
and God said
Let there be light
and there was light.

Ann Craig
Age 14
(DIARY ENTRY, AUGUST 1966)

Coming Home

On August 15, Dr. Evans asked me to meet him in the lobby of the hospital. We walked to the coffee shop together and sat at the busy counter.

"Ann's bleeding is under control now. She's stabilized on the AZT. She can go home if you are prepared to take her."

Suddenly I was frightened. "What if she bleeds again? How can I protect the rest of the family?"

"Separate sheets and towels. Clorox bleach in her laundry. Rubber gloves if she's bleeding. As long as your water runs hot she can use the silverware and dishes you use."

"When will you discharge her?" I asked.

"Take her tomorrow. Before she has another setback." Dr. Evans swiveled to face me fully. "From now on, every hour must stand for a day." His sad eyes searched my own. "And every day for a year."

"Should I stop working to be home with her?" I asked.

"Not yet," the doctor said. "You'll know when it's time to do that."

"Will you continue to take care of her?" I did not want Annie to lose Dr. Evans, but we lived thirty miles from his office.

"You'll be able to bring her to me. I'll see her every Monday after office hours, starting at six o'clock a week from next Monday."

"Dr. Evans, I wish I could thank the stranger I spoke to on the Gay Men's Hot Line in New Haven, who gave your name to me. Your kindness helps so much. I have just one last question. When did you know that Ann had AIDS?"

"The moment I saw her. In fact, the day you came to tell me about her I was certain," he said.

We finished a second cup of coffee and paid the blue-haired cashier. I put my hand on his arm as we walked back to the lobby. "Good luck with all that you're doing, Dr. Evans. If there's some way I could help, I would like to."

"There are just so many of them." He clapped his hand to his chest as though stricken with sudden pain. "I had to tell two more today. Tonight they'll be crying with their loved ones, and I'll be crying for them. We're keeping them alive longer with the AZT now. Long enough for some to go blind or suffer greater neurological impairment. So many, and some only little children. Yesterday we lost a three-year-old. Her mother had died last year."

He walked me to the elevator lobby, then clasped my hand in his own. "Good luck with our Annie," he said. "I'm glad she'll get to go home."

"Of course, she can come home," Paul said, but his face blanched as perhaps my own had when Dr. Evans told me.

"I'll shop tomorrow for separate dishes and glasses for her, as well as sheets and towels. I'll also call the Visiting Nurses Association and ask them to send help right away," I said.

That evening I was in the shower at 11:30 when Paul called out from the bed, "Hospital on the phone."

Ann had a raging fever. One hundred five degrees. I drove to the hospital and sat in a chair by her bed for the rest of the night while she received four lines of fluid through the shunt in her chest.

I was not sure she knew I was beside her, but sometime before

sunrise she murmured, "Mamma, I don't want to be smithereened."

"I wouldn't let that happen, Annie."

"I hope you won't be smithereened, either," she said, but she
did not open her eyes.

In the morning, with the fever down to 101, she asked me to
bring coffee and muffins from the little shop in the hospital lobby.
I had my breakfast at her bedside. She broke off a few bits of
crust from the edge of the muffin but left them on the cardboard
plate. She fell asleep with the coffee lid unopened.

Dr. Evans added four more days to Ann's hospitalization, "to
build her up as much as we can." Four days during which I set
up a kitchen in Ann's room. Our beachside cottage has two bed-
rooms and two baths on the second floor. I would put Ann in
the room behind ours, so I would hear her if she needed me.

I bought a microwave oven, a hot plate and blender, borrowed
a small refrigerator, and had cable TV installed. I hung a new
lace curtain on the window by her bed and a long one inside the
door that led to a little outside deck.

Two visiting nurses, who would supervise help for Ann at
home, went to see her in the hospital.

"How can we help you make the best adjustment from hospital
to home?" the head nurse asked.

"I do not really need any help," Ann said. "My mother doesn't
think I can stay alone while she's working. We just need someone
long enough for Mom to realize that I will be fine by myself."

"Okay," the visiting nurse said. "Why don't we go ahead and
plan for an interim person to be with you at home every day
until we reassess your needs?"

Release time was set for Friday at one o'clock. Thursday evening Paul took a call from a neighborhood couple whose son had
gone to school with Ann. They insisted on coming over, although I had a car full of glasses, dishes, and microwave-ware to
unload and set up.

"I don't feel like seeing anyone," I said. But Paul was already
putting ice in four glasses.

"Maybe they want to ask how they might be able to help," he said.

"Ed and I believe we have a right to be open." Marge Brewer sat next to me at the wrought-iron picnic table on the deck. "We feel we have a right to ask exactly what opportunistic diseases Ann might be carrying."

I began to answer politely, responsive to the fears she presented. Denying that I felt attacked.

"Will Ann be walking in the neighborhood?" Ed Brewer interrupted nervously. "Will you let her go to the beach?"

"By the way," his wife interrupted, "have you been tested yourself?"

"I have taken no risks with my own health. And I intend to take none," I said.

"We won't be dropping over while she's with you," his wife said. "Especially since our grandchildren will be with us Labor Day weekend."

I glanced at Paul, who looked as pleasant as he might during any social interaction.

"No, do not come over," I stood up. "Ann will be here. People who are uncomfortable with that will need to keep their distance. Excuse me. I have to fix up her room. It is Ann's time to be home now."

On Friday, August 13, as I was about to leave for the hospital, I took an urgent phone call from a client. She had opened a letter addressed to her husband and discovered that he was HIV positive. Hearing this woman cry, setting up a time for her, kept me late for Ann.

She was waiting in the wheelchair. She'd outlined her eyes with mascara. Her cheeks were softly rouged, lips glossy, her head wrapped in a ruby-colored turban with a rhinestone clasp on the side.

"How do you like our glamour girl?" Kathy asked.

"Well enough to think we ought to hit all the hot spots from Danbury to Westport." I bent to kiss her.

"I'll settle for a coffee milk shake," Annie grinned.

Kathy helped me pack the six baskets and four glass vases of silk and dried flower arrangements into two big cartons. In clearing off the windowsill, I found a basket of faded roses and started to throw away the shriveled flowers.

"Please save them, Mom," Ann pleaded.

Flooded with memories from eleven years before, vivid images of packing Ann's belongings at Austen Riggs, I put the dead flowers in a brown paper bag.

It took four trips from the tenth floor to the parking lot to load the car with the bags, boxes, books, nightgowns and bed jackets, turbans and sweaters accumulated in her three months at the hospital. Even from her sickbed Annie was a champion collector.

"Doctor sent prescriptions for her medication down to the pharmacy," Kathy said as I wheeled my daughter past the nurses' station. "And here's some information," Kathy handed Ann a packet of folders. Ann glanced at the collection of pamphlets, and held out the one titled: "What to Do When a Friend Has AIDS."

In big letters she wrote: "SHOOT HIM."

"Good-bye, Annie." "We'll miss you." Nurses, aides, even patients from their beds waved us down the hall.

"Thank you. Thanks for everything!" Ann called.

The pharmacy was on the emergency room level. We waited half an hour for the pharmacist to complete preparing her prescriptions. I had brought $100. With AZT the bill for ten days' medication came to $814. We had to wait the two long hours it took to have the smaller amounts of medication rebottled to amounts I could afford.

By the time we got home, Ann was exhausted. The aide the visiting nurse had sent, wide-eyed with fear about her first AIDS case, met us in the driveway. Ann walked to the front of the house to watch the sun set behind the harbor.

"Where she be at? What she doin' now?" the woman shrilled frantically.

"Ma," Ann glared at me, "I'll be leaving right away if she is going to be on my case like that."

I called the nurse supervisor, who thought that Ann and Yolanda would get used to one another. I said I doubted that was possible. Two days later the nurse supervisor sent Hattie, the same home health aide who had cared for John Coffee, the young client I had had who had died of AIDS. I knew how much Hattie meant to John. I watched hopefully as she introduced herself to Ann out on the deck.

"Hi, Annie," her voice was husky. "My name is Hattie. But everybody call me Cat."

"Listen, Cat," Ann scowled, "I do not need any help from anyone. If you think you have to be here, I want you to keep away from me and stay just long enough to prove to my mother that I can take care of myself."

"Well, now, I'm so glad to hear that!" Cat settled her generous body in a chair some distance from Ann. " 'Cause I just hate to work."

"And you better move further away." Ann bent to light a cigarette, cupping her hands to protect the flame from the gentle August breeze. "I smoke these powerful clove cigarettes all the time."

"Well, now, I'd just love to try me one of them fancy cigarettes." Cat went to Ann and reached out her hand.

Ann glanced at Cat's gleaming face, then slowly placed a cigarette on her palm.

From that day on, Ann and Cat spent hours on the deck together, smoking and swapping stories. Cat told sad ones about her life in Bridgeport, Connecticut. About her brother who was killed. About his son and the daughter she was raising alone. Hard, courageous, sometimes funny stories.

From my room above the deck I heard Cat ask Ann, "Tell me again, 'bout that black man got killed and how you went right to the mayor."

"I didn't go alone." I listened as Ann told Cat the story of how her friend Michael Stewart had been in the Pyramid Club on September 15, 1983. "You would have loved him, Cat. He was a wonderful artist and the nicest, gentlest man."

"I'm still lookin' to find me one of them," Cat said.

"Michael was arrested in the subway that night for putting graffiti on the station wall. They brought him to the hospital hog-tied and beaten. He died after thirteen days. The chief medical examiner lied, Cat. He said Michael was drunk. We all knew that wasn't true. He said there was no evidence that physical injury led to his death. That's why we went to the mayor. Later on the medical examiner lost his job."

"I'm proud you helped one a my people," Cat said.

Heading off to work, I could hear them laughing at a different Annie story, about the woman in the apartment beside hers, who kept over forty dogs. "And anytime anyone walked by the apartment, it set off all those dogs. But Effie, the woman, always barked the loudest. Like this," Annie yowled.

The Moon Is Broken

In her first two weeks at home Ann insisted on doing things that seemed impossible, given her terrifying frailty. Three times she went to the beach to swim. David took her out to dinner. Paul and I took her for a coffee ice cream soda at Baskin-Robbins. Just as we placed it in her hands, a tremor swept through her body and the frosty treat poured onto the pavement.

One week after her discharge from the hospital I drove her back to Dr. Evans's office for a checkup. For once, instead of insisting on privacy, Ann invited me to join her in his office. Clearly she trusted and loved this gentle, witty man.

"Tell my mamma I'll be ready to head back to the city soon," she prodded.

"Our star is doing so well I'm not even going to bother doing blood tests," he hugged her. "But Annie, between you and me, please don't run away from your mamma yet. I think she needs you to be with her for a little longer."

Driving home we decided to celebrate. I pulled into the roadhouse cocktail lounge Ann spotted. Hidden away from the boisterous bar crowd, over frosty piña coladas, we told each other our dreams. She wondered what her life would have been like if she had married Tim. I told her how I had taken the job at the prison, hoping to understand more about heroin from female users and how someday I hoped to write a play about the women I had worked with.

"I bet you will, Ma," she said enthusiastically. We grinned at each other. "Think I smile like you yet?" she asked.

"Exactly the same way," I said.

We ordered another round of piña coladas. I guzzled mine. Ann sipped at hers.

"I don't think I ever told you about the time I liberated the all-men's bar in New York City," she said. "Went there every night for a week before anyone would serve me. When I finally got to order, all I had in mind was a Coke. All the men banged on the bar and made jokes, that a woman invaded McSorley's for a Coca-Cola."

We laughed and then there was a silence before Ann spoke again. "There's something else I'd like to talk about, Ma. David is so angry at me and I don't know how I can help him. He is not angry out in the open. He is angry silently. Angry because I am dying. And I feel as though I can hear him saying, 'What about *me*, Ann? What am I supposed to do, Ann?' "

"Annie, you have to trust that David could learn how to go on without you, just as we would all find ways to be alone if we had to."

"It's not the same, Ma." She shook her head. "Will you promise to do me a favor? It's about David. Someday, would you buy him a beautiful T-shirt, really good quality, I mean, and have it printed with great big letters that say THINK BIG. And tell him it's from Ann."

"I promise." I smiled.

"And get the new babies special presents. I saved some ads I want to show you about baby furniture. When they can understand, tell them Aunt Ann never met them but she loved them."

Ann went on to name each person in the family, Ellen and Charlie, Richard and Rosemary, Bill and Nicola, her grandmother, her father, each of the stepsiblings and their wives— Andrew and Bettyann, Alex, Doug and Trisha, Kathy and Peter—all her aunts, uncles, and cousins and suggested gifts for each one. I took my grocery shopping notebook from my pocketbook and recorded her instructions.

Some of the relatives had not seen Ann in years. She was making peace with everyone. She was again the thoughtful person she had been as a child, never wanting anyone left out. Saying good-bye by taking care of others.

When Ann made her way to the bathroom, I watched people stare and nudge one another, commenting on her thinness. I had a fleeting wish to stand up on the table and scream at them. Help me! Don't just sit there staring when you can clearly see how sick she is.

The waitress came to pick up empty glasses. "I noticed how nice you are to that person," she said curiously.

"That person is my daughter," I said.

Driving home we stopped at the same spot by the reservoir where we paused the day I drove her to the hospital. Now reflected moonlight shimmered across the surface of the inky water.

"I'm glad we covered so many topics tonight, Ma."

"I am too. I feel so very close to you."

"There's one more thing I wanted to tell you."

"What is it, Annie?"

"I—I always hoped someday that I would have a baby. When I was in the psychiatric unit at the Yale–New Haven Hospital the resident doctor there told me I would always be infertile. I wasn't having periods then. I think some part of me gave up way back then, Mom, about ever having a normal kind of life."

"Annie, how come you never told me that before?" I wondered how any doctor could have been so certain. I knew many anorectic patients who recovered and bore children. Could Ann have misunderstood the doctor?

"I knew it would make you sad, Ma. That's why I didn't tell you. I never wanted to make you sad. But I decided then that I would never marry. Never have a baby. Never have a baby, Mom," she repeated.

"I am so sorry, Annie." I saw that her fingers were bleeding again. I pulled a rubber glove from my pocket and slipped it on to hold her hand the rest of our ride home together.

Ann was still asleep when Ellen brought little Charlie over to see her at nine the following morning. Charlie built towers with blocks in the living room as Ellen and I lingered over coffee at the kitchen table.

Her second child was due in just two months. "I wish it were a happier pregnancy for you, dear," I said.

"For Nicola, too," Ellen nodded. She and Billy's wife had due dates two weeks apart. Nicola was spending day after day in Vermont at the bedside of her father who was terminally ill with cancer.

"Last night I had the most vivid dream," Ellen sighed. "You and I were in your car trying to make our way through some kind of chaotic scene to get back home together. But a marriage procession was passing and we could not get beyond it. The bride and groom had started off together but suddenly she was going one way and the groom then headed off in the opposite direction. Then just in front of you and me a big black hearse pulled out and followed right behind the bride."

Little Charlie may have heard our sniffles. He came into the kitchen and crawled up on his mother's lap. "How will the baby get out?" He tapped her stomach, then sucked on his finger.

"Didn't we just talk about that last night?" She kissed his auburn hair, so like her own, and smiled at me through bleary eyes.

The last days of August were hot and humid. Ann needed lighter clothes. She especially asked for white pleated shorts with pockets. We went shopping in a local store. I planned to buy her anything she wanted. Ann checked the clothes racks while I went to the counter to ask where shorts might be found. But the saleswoman said all the summer merchandise had been shipped to another store.

I turned, but could not find Ann to tell her. I felt the same wave of panic experienced so many years ago when, as a little girl, she once had wandered off in a supermarket. Then I found her, sitting under a rack of dresses, too tired to look for anything.

In our absence Cat had placed the morning mail on the kitchen counter. There was a package for Ann, return address Los Angeles.

"Can you believe it!" she said. "Randy sent me exactly what I was looking for today. We really have some kind of psychic connection." She held his gift against her wasted body. White pleated shorts with pockets.

Ann spent that Friday afternoon planning a party for Cat, whose birthday was just three days away. With her vision continuing to deteriorate, she had to use a thick felt marker to write and rewrite lists of guests, possible menus, a plan for the "stakeout" to surprise Cat, even the beginnings of a script for entertainment.

But Ann began to sleep more often. She was less alert when she wakened. The day before the party she wanted to buy favors at the drugstore. I had barely driven down the road that brilliant balmy afternoon when her head drooped to the side. Frightened, I called her name. I was relieved when she murmured.

I drove back home. Paul helped me get her to bed. We placed a call to Dr. Evans.

"She's becoming very weak again."

"Can you manage her at home?" he asked. "Would you rather have her in the hospital?"

I remembered the times her mind and body seemed beyond revival. Yet within hours of blood transfusions, intravenous feedings, tubes, and shots, she would be alert again.

"You would not want to take heroic measures," Dr. Evans addressed the thoughts I had not spoken. "Her eyesight is rapidly failing. Intervention cannot change that. Her last laboratory tests before she left the hospital defied her being alive even then. That's why I didn't bother drawing blood in my office. Each scan shows more profoundly how the virus is attacking her brain. . . ."

"Then she will stay at home," I said.

Reviving her again would be only for me. Not for Annie.

Randy called that evening. It was his birthday. He had to speak to Annie. She was too weak to hold the phone. I held the receiver to her ear.

"Oh, Eleanor," Randy spoke to me afterward. "I hear how feeble she sounds. Please I beg you, can you put her on a plane? I can take her with me to Mexico. There's going to be a new beginning, Eleanor! The powerful Harmonic Conversions. The end of the century. Do you know about it? The Aztecs and the Mayans saw it coming. The planetary alliance. It is now the Age of the Sixth Sun. It *was* the age of the Fifth Sun. Oh, can you understand the healing power? I beg you, let Annie come to Mexico with me now. I need to be with the person who taught me all I know. I've taken all the tools and knowledge she has given me. It is my turn to help her now. New life! New beginning! It will give her healing powers. Oh, can you understand it, Eleanor? An astroflash from God!"

"I understand, Randy. Annie is too sick to be moved. I know she would have loved to see an astroflash from God."

Ann stayed in her room on Monday. She could not eat the soup that Cat made for her, but took some sips of soda from a tablespoon.

"Cat," she clutched her new friend's arm, "I want a beautiful stone."

"Now that's a fine way to be thinkin' on my birthday, Annie honey."

"Happy Birthday, Cat." Ann made a kiss sound and closed her eyes.

"Your mamma gonna get your stone." Cat gently rearranged the blankets.

At eleven that night I gave up on sleep and spent the next three hours at the kitchen table, fitfully reading *Dinner at the Homesick Restaurant*—the story of the family that never quite fulfills the fantasy of just one perfect meal together. Too tired to read any longer, too anxious to close my eyes, I spotted the yellow folder I had prepared for Ann. The night I took it to the hospital she had been too weak to look.

I sorted through the contents. Baby pictures of Ann. The yellowed newspaper article quoting her description of art at the age of six.

> *Art is a piece of imagination*
> *Art is seeing things in your own way*
> *and painting them that way in colors you like.*

Art is something that can tell a story.
Art is a language all its own. It has no letters.
Art is something most people love.

A glossy photo of Ann in her ninth grade prom dress, with Alan Spiegel half a head shorter than she, holding the corsage box. The note she wrote at fourteen to her father, who was in Japan, working on his first book.

> Dear King,
> We all miss you. I notice that you even write letters like an author. If I shut my eyes, I could see them in a Readers' Digest article—"A Famous Father's Letters to His Family." But we'd rather have you home than receive the beautiful letters.
> Please come back soon.
>
> Your devoted daughter,
Ann
>
> P.S. Watch out for them geisha's, y'hear?

A picture from the Brown alumni magazine of Annie making a dulcimer. Letters from Africa. Write-ups from *The New York Times* about the Pyramid Club. . . .

Suddenly I heard a creaking sound. It grew more distracting. Was it from the ceiling or the cupboards? Could some small animal be trapped?

As I got up to investigate I was startled by Ann's sudden appearance at the bottom of the stairway. She had crept down the steps to keep from falling. "I—I—could not—sleep—either—Mom."

I helped her to a chair and made us both hot chocolate. Then I pulled her chair next to mine and we went through the collection of memorabilia together. She stared at a five-by-seven photograph of herself about ten, with Richard, Billy, and little Ellen who was only two.

"Some—somehow—" she said haltingly, "we've all had such a—spiritual connection."

"We always will." I had my arm around her. Then like a little child, she crawled into my lap.

"Mamma." She touched my cheek. Her eyes were fearful. "Have

I done something wrong? Do, do I deserve to be punished? I mean by God, Ma."

"Annie, how could there be a God who would not love and understand you? All I can say to you about your suffering is that if I get to meet Him, He's going to have to answer lots of questions."

I tucked her into bed reciting the nighttime poem from her childhood. Annie whispered with me:

> *Good night*
> *Good night*
> *Far flies the light*
> *And still God's love*
> *Shall shine above*
> *Making all bright.*
> *Good night. Good night.*

An hour later Ann fell out of bed. She groaned with pain. Dr. Evans ordered morphine.

A neighbor nurse showed me how to administer the shots. I was terrified to do it, but my need to reduce her pain far outweighed my hesitation.

Annie, here's another shot for you. And I called the priest for you too, dear. Father Driscoll will be here tomorrow. He will give you Last Rites.

Father Driscoll anointed her body, administering the final sacrament of the Catholic faith.

Dr. Robbins also came to the house.

"Have I done something wrong?" she murmured.

"I always think of how hard you tried, Ann," her first psychiatrist answered. "You never wanted to hurt others. You were always very special to me."

She smiled and closed her eyes.

Wednesday night Ellen brought little Charlie over for me to watch. She had come to say good-bye to her sister.

Although it was 9:00 P.M., I took my little grandson for a walk toward the beach.

"Mommy said the doctor can't fix Annie, Bamma," he slipped his hand in mine. "No doctors couldn't fix her either. They tried. The hossible couldn't fix her either. The hossible tried. And you tried too. But she has EEDS."

"Yes, it is a terrible disease."

"Annie did drugs," little Charlie sighed. "But Annie was a friend to everyone. Annie loved me so much."

Charlie spoke of Ann in past tense. "She does love you so much—" I said.

"Oh no, Bamma!" he interrupted, pointing. "Oh no! Look! See? The moon is broken!"

I picked up my grandson and we both gazed up at the crescent moon. "It isn't really broken, dear. The whole moon is always there, but we can't always see it. I'll tell you a moon poem Annie used to like.

> *Dear mother, how pretty*
> *The moon looks tonight*
> *She was never so cunning before:*
> *Her two little horns*
> *Are so sharp and so bright*
> *I hope she'll not grow any more."*

As I carried Charlie home, a sweet sound filtered from Ann's open bedroom window. Ann, in a wavering voice, made the tick-tock sound as Ellie more firmly sang the words . . .

> *My grandfather's clock*
> *Was too large for the shelf . . .*

Then Ann's voice strengthened as she finished the song with her sister:

> *But it stopped—short—*
> *Never—to—go—again—*
> *When the old man died.*

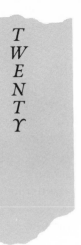

Now It's Time
to Say Good-bye

Two weeks after she came home, I saw that my Annie was dying. We sent for her father, who was still living in the Virgin Islands. Billy arrived from New Hampshire and took turns with me administering her morphine. At night he slept on a mat by her bed. By day, Ellen, David, and I kept vigil.

On Thursday morning she said good-bye to me.

"You will be with me always. All the rest of my life. Every day. You will be with me." I held her.

"I fixed the flowers," she pointed feebly. "Please don't touch the flowers."

Moments later my watch stopped.

Ellen brought a tape recorder for Ann to hear the beautiful sea sounds she loved. In the middle of the second playing of the tape, the new recorder broke. No amount of fixing could make it play again.

Big, gentle David never left her side, watching, waiting hour after hour. Thursday night the hospice group sent a young man who expected to be able to talk with Ann. Seeing her semi-comatose, he chose to stay and sit beside her bed with David.

"Ann wanted me to promise," David told the hospice volunteer, "that when this time arrived I would give her shots or pills to keep her from having to linger."

"Then you must be wondering what to do now," the young stranger nodded. "People who love her have to trust her also. She will know when to go."

I thought I ought to let Tim know how limited Ann's time was. But I did not want to hurt David's feelings, so I asked if he would mind my calling Tim.

"Surely call him," David said. "I know how much he meant to Ann."

Tim was writing filmscripts. I dialed his New York apartment, half expecting the recorded message giving his telephone number in California. But Tim answered the phone at 11:00 P.M., and responded by renting a car. He arrived in Westport at 2:00 A.M.

Friday morning I woke up with a strong feeling that I must wear something pink and dress Ann in pink as well. Up to now, for convenience, Cat and I had kept her in the yellow cotton hospital gowns. I put on my pink sweater, and went to Annie's room to look for something pink for her. But Cat had already dressed her in a pink silk gown.

"Somehow, I thought it would ease our Annie's passing if we dress her up today," Cat said. "Seem like she oughta be in pink."

By the time of her father's arrival, Ann was too comatose to be responsive. But she had left each of us with a message. I felt sad for Bill that it was too late for him to have a final chance to hear her voice.

The family kept a silent vigil. The priest came by to pray for her. I sat by her head telling her not to be afraid, that it would be more beautiful than any of us could ever imagine. At two o'clock on Friday afternoon Billy whispered to me, "If I were dying and you were holding on to my hand and talking like that to me, Mother, I would not be able to leave you either."

We began taking silent turns at her bedside. At half past six, her father asked for time alone. He sang to her the Irish lullabye he used to sing when she was a baby.

Toora loora loora—
Hush now don't you cry. . . .

"Daddy?" Ann murmured. And then her breathing changed.

Bill called us back to the room.
"Annie, we love you!"
"Good-bye! Good-bye!" we cried.
"Go to the light, dear Annie. Stay with the light."
"You will be with us—always."
"Annie, I brought your beautiful stone," Tim called. "The one we got in Ethiopia."
Tim placed the stone in my hand. I wrapped Ann's fingers around the African stone.
"We love you, Annie! We love you!"
Annie exhaled. She did not take another breath.

Cat and I wrapped her body in her pink flowered sheet. We all waited at the bottom of the stairs as they carried Annie down.
Then we stood in the driveway waving and calling good-bye. One last Irish Good-bye. I closed my eyes until the hearse was out of sight.

Epilogue: Letting Go

Ellen, round with child, stood before the crowd at Ann's memorial service to read the poem she'd written for her sister:

> For Ann
> Whose each dream defied imagining
> And was greater
> than the most solid fantasies.
> For Annie, who signed her
> name with a star . . .

Then Billy gave his eulogy.

It was impossible not to love Annie. Anyone who spent a minute with her was fascinated; anyone who enjoyed an hour of her matchless company was smitten. She lifted hearts. She gave us glimpses of a powerful esthetic, shared her astonishing knowledge and experience, dazzled us. Over and over, one and all, we fell in love with her.

But loving Annie was not always easy. Her vulnerability, her danger frightened us; her illness and her anger grieved us. We didn't understand. We couldn't make her better. To love her so and let go again and again—this wasn't easy. We would have given anything to help her, but Annie would not take. Instead she gave all she could, whenever she was able. Time and again she gave me back double the life I wanted to give her. It wasn't always easy loving Annie, but I know it will be much harder to live without her. . . .

A friend sang "Let It Be."

For me the grieving came in waves. Driving, I sometimes had to pull to the side of the road to give vent to the tears. At home I began to arrange a shrine. I spread Annie's photographs across the fireplace mantel. I framed the Coptic art she had sent from Africa. The silk flowers from her room at the hospital, which she had laced with strings of pearl and crystal beads, adorned her bureau exactly as she'd left them. I kept her leather jacket, sequined sweaters, her paisley shawl in her closet.

As fate would have it, the Child Guidance Center referred a child to me whose mother had died of cancer. The eight-year-old did not see her mother after she entered the hospital for the last time. With dolls, the child revealed to me all the reasons why her mother could have gone away. She might have had to visit a friend. Or go on a long vacation. Then she played out their reunion.

I, too, comforted myself with magical thinking. Ann had so often absented herself, only to reappear in our lives. Mornings, on my way to work, I paused by the door to her room as though there might still be one more good-bye.

Two months after Annie's death, Ellen gave birth to Paulina. On that very day, Billy called from New Hampshire to announce the birth of baby Anne. That night I dreamed of telling Annie about the same-day births of her nieces. "Irish twins." She laughed. "Give them both a kiss for me."

In December clients spoke of holidays being too painful to acknowledge, even after losses that occurred many years before. I asked Paul to help me to enhance, rather than diminish, our

Christmas/Channukah observations. For Annie, we added more lights to the tree.

We survivors had drawn even closer. Ellen and I met weekly with a hospice worker. We took a trip to Hong Kong to see Richie and his family. Billy and I stayed in frequent contact.

I also kept in touch with Ann's friends. David plunged into a long, creative period of painting. Tim's filmscript won a prize in Europe.

"I feel her star power beaming down on me," Randy said. "That woman. That crone. That beautiful spirit. What a blessing. What a curse to have been born with so much energy. Your daughter was a channel, Eleanor. She could pull it out of everyone. She just could not live with it herself."

As the first year passed, the intensity of pain never lessened. But gradually it came less often. And even more slowly, in its place I began to feel a deep resolve to live the rest of my life as fully as I could, empowered by the strength I had been forced to realize in having had to survive the loss of a child.

One afternoon, I watched as my eight-year-old client was playing with the dollhouse in my office. She put the mother on the rooftop near the chimney. Down in the kitchen she sat the girl doll and the father across from an empty chair. Then she backed away to study the scene.

"At first when you died," she reached for the mother doll and shook her, "I couldn't find my shoes or anything. And I was mad. You broke your promise that you wouldn't go away. But now," she held the mother to her cheek, "I feel as if you're always with me. Like the wind is. Even though I only get to see you when I dream."

That night, I undid my shrine. I put away all but Ann's most recent photograph, and surrounded that with pictures of all my children and stepchildren. I packed her clothes for the homeless and rearranged her room.

I was half awake, half dreaming. "Annie," I said, "it's time for me to let go. I know that you are at peace now. I want to hold to you with love, instead of with sadness. Then we can both be free."

"Well, thank goodness, Ma." She nodded as though I had at last agreed to her suggestion. "I was wondering when you'd get around to doing that. And remember, what I said to Richie goes for all the rest of you. Please. For me. Keep fun in your hearts."

Afterword

At first, I wasn't really sure if I could write an afterword for *The Moon Is Broken*. But after reading Eleanor Craig's book, I thought that no one knows better than I what she might have felt or thought, for I had gone through a bitter experience like hers. *The Moon Is Broken* expresses what mothers everywhere love about and fear for their children. And no matter how young or old, when your child dies, the pain and loss are always the same.

Like Eleanor, I was the mother unable to help soothe the hurts, make things right. I felt as if it was my hand holding Annie's. It broke my heart to relive with Eleanor the fevers, the loss of appetite and weight. Annie was so full of life, always wanting to help someone else, ease someone else's burden, protect someone else from pain or worry. I can't tell you how many times I cried when Eleanor told of Annie's experiences in the mental hospitals. Why this beautiful and loving child was unable to share her grief over the terrible tragedy of rape with her mother, I don't know. What I do know that you make sure you do your very best in bringing up your children to feel loved and cared for and then you set them free and hope you've done everything right.

I was lucky in that Ryan was always there with me, so I could look after his every need. Eleanor was not that fortunate. It would have torn my heart out not knowing where my child was—on the brink of death somewhere in New York City, alone. Sometimes the words of other parents who have lost a child help you to realize you are not alone, that there are many others who have gone through this kind of experience and have learned not to blame themselves. Until people experience the death of a child, I'm not sure they realize the strength it takes to move on to the next day.

When I finished reading Annie's story, I cried for Ryan, and then I thanked God for my children. I thought, I want to hold Andrea, my own beloved daughter, as close to my heart as possible. But as Annie's story shows, you have to set your children free—to choose what's best for themselves, no matter how much it might hurt or worry you. Then, if they've chosen a rocky path, you must be there to pick up the pieces and try to make things right again.

I truly believe that every day that passes, Ryan, from where he is now, is helping me understand and accept the events that happened in our lives. It may sound silly, but I believe he is watching over his family still. And Annie, too—through this book—will touch so many people. She is now in a place where she can do things to help, once again, the ones she loved and left behind. So, as Annie would say, "Don't worry, Ma. I am alright!"

Mrs. Jeanne White,
mother of Ryan White
September 1991